Contents

Acknowledgements

I'd like to thank the various people at Nelson Thornes who have collaborated with me on this text; the many health care students and teachers with whom I have worked, particularly Sheri, Steffe and Trish; and Lynne Wigens who has offered unconditional help and support throughout the project. I would also like to thank the students and health care professionals who have contributed their experiences to the text, especially Dave Oakley, whose comments were gratefully received.

'Patients Reunited' reprinted courtesy of Take a Break magazine.

'Communications guidelines from the Royal College of Surgeons' copyright © the Royal College of Surgeons of England. Reproduced with permission. The full text of this document can be found at www.rcseng.ac.uk/services/publications/publications/pdf/gsp2002.pdf

Health belief model information. Reprinted from the Journal of Clinical Epidemiology volume **49**(6):697–703, Mezaros et al. Rahe, 'Cognitive processes and the decisions of some parents to forego pertussis vaccination for their children', copyright © 1996, with permission from Elsevier.

Extract from *Our Healthier Nation* © Crown copyright. Crown copyright material is reproduced with the permission of the Controller of HMSO and the Queen's Printer for Scotland.

'Poor recall mars research and treatment' by Beth Azar, reprinted from the APA Monitor, January 1997, copyright © American Psychological Association. Permission applied for.

'Sisters can do it for themselves' by Rebecca Hardy. Reprinted with permission from the Independent Review, 12th January 2004.

'Stop or you won't see your children grow up' reprinted courtesy of Take a Break magazine.

'I get a lot more kissing now I've quit' reprinted courtesy of Take a Break magazine.

'The Social Readjustment Rating Scale' reprinted from the Journal of Psychosomatic Research Volume 11, Holmes and Rahe, pages 213–218, copyright © 1967, with permission from Elsevier.

Foundations in Nursing and Health Care

Introduction to Psychology for Health Carers

Julia Russell

Series Editor: Lynne Wigens

Published in 2005 by:
Nelson Thornes Ltd
Delta Place
27 Bath Road
CHELTENHAM
GL53 7TH
United Kingdom

05 06 07 08 09 / 10 9 8 7 6 5 4 3 2 1

A catalogue record for this book is available from the British Library

ISBN 0 7487 8074 2

Illustrations by Clinton Banbury
Page make-up by Florence Production Ltd, Stoodleigh, Devon

Printed in Great Britain by Ashford Colour Press

'Use a big stick to beat stress' by Judith Woods copyright ©
    Telegraph Group Limited 2003
'Coping with stress' copyright © the Royal College of Psychiatrists.
    Reproduced with permission. The full text of this document can
    be found at www.rcpsych.ac.uk/info/mhgu/newmhgu32.htm
'What is stress?' 'Why stress matters' and 'What can give rise to
    stress at work?' copyright © the Mental Health Foundation.
    Reproduced with permission.
'Symptoms of stress' reprinted with kind permission of NHS Health
    Scotland.
'It's true: a healthy mind can cure' by Anthony Browne copyright ©
    Guardian Newspapers Limited 2001.

Photographs

Soldier injured. Corel 759 (NT)
Sportsperson/injury, Photodisc 40 (NT)
'A nerve cell and synapse' (P360/181) copyright © David Gifford/
    Science Photo Library

Every effort has been made to trace the copyright holders but if any
have been inadvertently overlooked, the publishers will be pleased to
make the necessary arrangement at the first opportunity.

Dedication

To Sheri with love, Julia

Preface

Health care professionals are in constant contact with other people: patients, their visitors and colleagues. The study of psychology – a scientific approach to the understanding of people's thinking and behaviour – can help to enhance the work of health carers. Whether you are just starting out on your career in health care, or are an established practitioner, this book will help you to understand some of the factors that influence people's decisions and actions. This knowledge will enable you to approach your work in a more professional and effective way.

The content of this book is divided into topics, such as 'communication' and 'stress'. In each chapter the topic is considered from the perspective of both the patient and the health care practitioner. This will enable you to gain insight into the issues facing your patients and to envisage ways in which you can improve your own practice.

The book was written after many years of teaching psychology to health care students at different levels. Psychology has many uses beyond the classroom and this text intends to show you how the findings of psychological research can help in the practical situations faced by health care professionals.

Julia Russell
October 2004

Introduction

The purpose of the book is to provide an introduction to psychology for students on health care courses, especially those who are returning to learning after a break or are in their first year of courses such as nursing or physiotherapy. It aims to present some of the key ideas in psychology that are relevant to health care settings, including those that are covered in the Foundation Degree in Health.

Each chapter has a range of features designed to help you to understand and apply the knowledge presented. All students tackling psychology for the first time are shocked because it uses a whole new vocabulary – it feels as though you are learning another language. To help you, all the specialist and important terms are defined under **keywords** in the margin and are described in more detail in the text. Keywords appear in bold the first time they are used within the text. To direct you, each chapter begins with a **learning framework**; you can use this to identify your aims as well as guiding you through the text. More complex ideas are summarised as **key points** and an overview of each chapter is presented in the **conclusions**. You will be encouraged to think about the new ideas and to test your understanding in the **over to you** sections, and **reflective activities** offer you the chance to see how the material you have been working on applies to the health care settings that you have experienced. To help you to visualise psychology in action in the health care environment, two further features, **students speaking** *and* **professionally speaking**, provide insight into the experiences of students on placement and qualified staff. Finally, **rapid recap** questions at the end of each chapter will provide you with a chance to test your knowledge. The answers are included at the back of the book.

Psychology uses many different techniques to explore human (and animal) thinking and behaviour. Theories – potential explanations – for different behaviours are examined by various kinds of research. This research may be based on artificial laboratory settings, in which experiments can be conducted and closely controlled, or in more naturalistic environments such as hospitals. Other research methods used in psychology include observations, questionnaires, interviews and case studies. Some examples of each of these are described. The evidence provided by research enables psychologists to refine their theories, hence there may be several alternative explanations for a single phenomenon. Each theory or piece of research is associated with a reference – a name (or names) and a date. These refer to the author and date of publication of the book or journal article in which the ideas appeared. It is important that you use these in your work. *Study Skills in Health Care* in this series will help you with this.

There are many ways in which psychology can help us to understand the behaviour, feelings and mental processing – such as beliefs and memory – of patients and health care professionals. When a person believes they may be ill they engage in activities called illness behaviours such as seeking – or avoiding – advice and treatment. We explore some of the psychological factors affecting the decision to seek help, for example personality (in Chapter 4) and health beliefs (in Chapter 2). Following diagnosis a patient demonstrates sick role behaviour, which assumes that being ill is not the patient's own fault, that they are freed (to an extent) from their day-to-day demands and that they will engage in activities in order to recover. At least some of the psychological evidence, however, suggests that people are surprisingly poor at accepting the sick role, for example by failing to follow advice (see Chapters 2 and 3).

There is a range of other ways in which psychology can inform health care practice. In Chapter 1, 'Communication in the health care setting', we consider the importance of communication in health care settings, exploring the various ways in which patients and practitioners interact and the advantages and disadvantages of different communication styles and other factors that influence the effectiveness of interactions.

Chapter 2, 'Explaining and changing health behaviour', begins by considering different explanations of people's health-related behaviour. The chapter goes on to discuss how those explanations can be used to understand the effectiveness of health promotion programmes and to suggest ways in which these could be improved.

In Chapter 3, 'Adherence to treatment', we explore why patients do or do not follow the medical advice they receive and consider ways to improve adherence to treatment. Explanations relating to attention, memory, thinking and behaviour are discussed.

'Stress', the title of Chapter 4, is important both to patients (as a cause or consequence of their ill-health) and to health care staff. In this chapter biological and psychological explanations of stress are described, as are factors that worsen, or help to alleviate, stress, including our own defences.

In Chapter 5, 'Pain', we investigate how pain has been explained and assess whether factors that affect the experience of pain, such as emotions, thinking and our behaviour, can be accounted for. The chapter concludes with a discussion of different approaches to pain relief.

Finally Chapter 6, 'Bereavement and grief', discusses the psychological effects of the death of a person we know well. A bereaved individual goes through a range of emotions and behaviours. These are described and individual differences in these responses are considered. The chapter ends by exploring ways in which recovery from the loss may be eased.

1

Communication in the health care setting

Learning outcomes

By the end of this chapter you should be able to:

- Recognise the roles of communication in the health care setting
- Discuss factors affecting successful spoken communication
- Explain the importance of non-spoken aspects of communication, such as non verbal communication and personal space
- Identify examples of good communication
- Identify examples of barriers to communication
- Evaluate interactions
- Describe psychological theories that help us to understand the communication process
- Apply these theories to health care settings
- Suggest ways to improve communication in health care settings
- Explain the need for confidentiality in successful, professional interaction.

In this chapter we explore the psychological factors that impact upon communication. Some communication issues are common to all settings, such as the value of listening as well as speaking or the importance of eye contact. In other ways, however, the health care setting is special. Patients may be less effective communicators for many reasons and adhering to conventions, such as those applying to invasion of personal space, may be impractical in some instances. It is precisely these issues that make effective communication so valuable. Even though health care workers such as nurses are constantly engaged with patients, much evidence suggests that their communication skills are insufficient to meet patient needs (Macleod Clark 1982).

We will consider a range of key variables in interactions, for example the use of jargon, the age of patients and the gender of the clinician, and consider the evidence suggesting that they are important in health care environments. The aim of the chapter is for you to be able to understand and recognise these factors in your own work and to evaluate the impact of your own **communication**.

What is communication?

Insel and Roth (1996, p. 86) define communication as 'the process by which we establish contact and exchange information with others'. This simple definition draws attention to many of the key issues in communication:

- Communication can only be effective if we have established contact – our audience must be paying attention or we will simply be ignored
- Communication is a process – it is not a single, simple act
- Communication requires an exchange – it is a two-way event.

⊶ᴛ *Keywords*

Communication
A two-way process of
interaction that is dependent
on the reception of, and
feedback in response to,
information

Establishing contact allows the initiator of the communication – the sender – to ensure that their message will be received. In a busy ward environment, or when dealing with patients whose communication skills are impaired, it is important to ensure that the receiver, the person for whom the message is intended, is going to see or hear the communication and will recognise that it is meant for them. Communication is a process, not a single act. Speaking, waving or clapping might be a signal but this only becomes communicative if it is part of an ongoing process – it must be received and acknowledged.

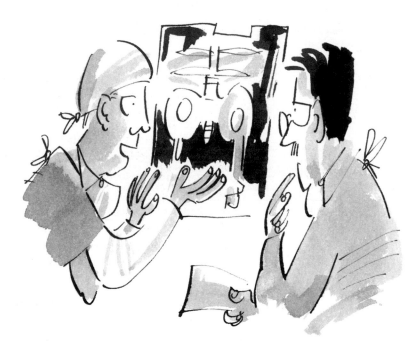

These two health care professionals are clearly identifiable from this event – it acts as a source of ritual information. In addition, their verbal conversation is accompanied by non-verbal messages, from eye contact, their clothing and their facial expressions

Information may be transmitted from sender to receiver using several communication channels or media. Stratton and Hayes (1988) identify three different routes:

- **Verbal** – using language or codes that stand for language, e.g. speech in a consultation or written patient records
- **Non-verbal** – the use of dress, posture, gesture or gaze, e.g. fear indicated by pacing in a waiting room or grief indicated by bereaved relatives wearing black

- **Ritual** – the use of highly structured events to communicate, e.g. a patient may communicate to a physiotherapist their level of movement by the range of specific tasks they can perform.

These communication channels may be used independently, for instance when we point to provide information (non-verbal) or receive a written note (verbal). Alternatively, and more commonly, they are used simultaneously, for example speech (verbal communication) is generally accompanied by non-verbal facial expressions.

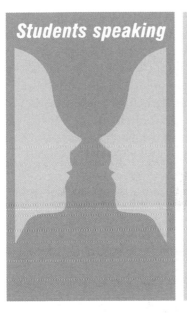

Students speaking

Communication and caring – the importance of explanations to patients

Student nurse on a surgical ward

Last week a patient was clerked in and he had signed a consent form for a TURP* I went over to him to help him get washed the next day, after the operation. He said 'Oh, I didn't realise that they would put a tube in there, and I didn't realise I'd have a drip. I thought they were going to cut me'. I said, 'Well did the doctor not explain to you when you were admitted?', and he said that if he had he had not taken it in. I said, 'Did you sign a consent form?' 'Oh yes', he said.

I think this happens quite frequently, probably because people are so nervous about having an operation, and perhaps they are too in awe of the consultant to ask any questions. So really it is important that informed consent is signed for after careful explanation and checking of understanding

* TURP Transurethral prostatectomy – removal of the prostate using the same urethral route as for urinary catheter insertion.

Exchange of information may be the primary goal of communication, such as when a nurse asks a patient to lift their arm to have their blood pressure taken. Alternatively, the exchange of information may be secondary, acting as a tool used by the sender to affect the state of the recipient, for example to reassure, coax, involve or empower patients or to provide mutual support between colleagues.

It is useful here to consider how communication is identified in animals. Krebs and Davies (1993, p. 349) define communication as 'the process in which actors [senders] use specifically designed signals or displays to modify the behaviour of reactors [recipients]'. This definition is helpful as it enables us to recognise that the purpose of communication is not solely to exchange information, but it may be an event in itself. Such non-exchange functions of communication are being identified as increasingly important and are probably a more significant factor in wellbeing than has previously been recognised.

In many situations, however, problems may arise with either exchange or non-exchange functions. For example, Ley (1988) analysed surveys of hospital patients and found that 41% felt that they had been given too little information, suggesting that the informational role of communication is often unsatisfactory. Patients may not understand or remember what they have been told, practitioners may be unable to obtain the information they require to ensure appropriate diagnosis or care and the supportive role of communication for both patients and staff may be inadequate.

Failures of communication may arise because practitioners and patients (or practitioners differing in status or discipline) enter into interactions with different agenda. The function of communication from a medical perspective is to diagnose and treat a biological pathology. Thus, communication primarily serves the function of information exchange to achieve the desired end point of effective treatment. For the patient, the primary reasons for communication may be personal, such as reassurance (e.g. Chaitchik *et al.* 1992). This discrepancy in function may account for instances such as misdiagnosis by doctors (lack of information from patients) and dissatisfied patients (lack of support from doctors). Neither communicator has fully achieved their goal because their intentions at the outset were different.

Over to you

Identify the medium used in each of the following examples of communication:

- health care professionals using formal clothing such as a uniform to indicate status or role
- A patient communicating their concerns by saying how they feel about having a general anaesthetic
- A student on placement signalling that they need help with a drip by making eye-contact with a qualified practitioner
- A visitor identifying an unfamiliar woman as a consultant because she is conducting a ward round.

⌕ₙ *Keywords*
···

Communication cycle
An interactive process between communicators that consists of messages being sent, received and responded to with feedback to the orginator of the message

The communication cycle

Communication involves the transmission of a message from one individual (the sender) to another (the recipient) but we can most readily understand communication as an *interactive* process if we consider the importance of a response from the recipient. The **communication cycle** completes the interaction with feedback from the recipient being received by the initial sender.

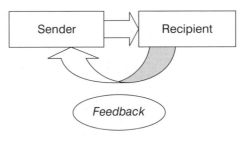

The communication cycle

Over to you

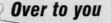

Communication failure can arise from a breakdown at any point in the communication cycle. Identify the point at which the cycle is broken in each of these instances:

● A nurse mumbles when she asks a patient a question

● A patient refuses to respond when prompted to express his anxieties about an operation

● A consultant isn't paying attention to a patient's comments about her treatment

● A student's reply to a question about a patient during a ward handover is interrupted by a contribution from another member of staff

● A patient cannot hear a question being asked about her symptoms.

Classifying communication

Communication in different circumstances, using different media and employed for different reasons, can be classified in a number of different ways. We have already discussed three communication processes or channels – verbal (which may be spoken or non-spoken), non-verbal and ritual communication (see pages 2–4) – and we will look at these in more detail later in the chapter. Interactions can also be classified as formal or informal. Formal communication involves individuals operating in their official capacity and tends to have an organised structure. This would include letters to patients describing procedures for admission to hospital or a case conference about a specific patient. Informal communication, in contrast, tends to be more relaxed and personal in nature, although individuals may still be acting in their formal role, such as nurses talking to patients as they attend to their dressings or wash their feet. Finally, interactions can be classified according to the number of participants, communication may be one-to-one, such as in a telephone call to a patient, or in a group, such as at a handover.

Table 1.1 Types of communication		
Communication medium	**Number of senders and/or recipients**	
Spoken	*One*	*Many*
	Patient to health care professional conversation Consultation Professional to professional appraisal	Meetings Case conferences Shift handovers on a ward
Non-verbal	Prescriptions Memos Referral letters	Minutes from meetings Patient records Service-user questionnaires

Why do we need to communicate in health care settings?

Communication can serve a host of different functions in the health care setting. Beckman *et al.* (1989) reviewed the outcomes or products of doctor–patient interactions and identified four distinct categories:

- **Process outcomes**. These occur during the medical encounter and include the elicitation of the patient's concerns and agreement about treatment options
- **Short-term outcomes**. These arise immediately after the medical encounter and include patient understanding, recall and intention to comply with advice, and doctor and patient satisfaction
- **Intermediate outcomes**. These are delayed until the patient is able to respond. They include the patient's actual compliance with advice, and changes in their anxiety, knowledge or self-esteem
- **Long-term outcomes**. The endpoint of treatment. These include quality of life, reduction of symptoms and survival.

Successful outcomes at each stage are important to the final resolution of health problems and many of these outcomes are determined, at least in part, by effective communication. For example, interruptions and the use of questions are important determinants of process outcomes as a measure of effective doctor–patient interactions (Beckman and Frankel 1984) and, as we will see in Chapter 3, patients' recall of the information they have been given affects their compliance with advice.

One key outcome, patient satisfaction, has proved difficult to study. Hall and Dornan have reviewed 221 studies of patient satisfaction and found that, despite considerable variation in the methods used, these studies report surprisingly consistent results, with about 40% of patients being dissatisfied with their treatment (Hall and Dornan 1988a, 1988b, 1990). Whilst there are issues about the reliability and validity of individual studies, such a finding is a poor reflection on the quality of care from the patients' perspective. Patient health is clearly a factor in patient satisfaction, although this also appears to be dependent upon the doctor's use of social conversation (Hall *et al.* 1998). This suggests that, even where there are clear medical issues, communication may play a significant role in patients' perception. Similarly, Daghio *et al.* (2003) found that doctor satisfaction was, in part, a function of good positive interactions with their patients and feeling professionally esteemed.

Reflective activity

Try to create a list of examples of communication being used for different functions in health care settings. Can you identify for each situation:

● The sender(s) and receiver(s)?

● Whether the situation is formal or informal?

● Whether it is a one-to-one or group setting?

● Whether the communication is predominantly verbal, non-verbal, ritual or mixed?

In each case, consider the purpose of the interaction for each sender and receiver.

In your list you have probably found a wide range of functions for communication. These functions can be divided into two broad categories:

● **Informational communication** – to transmit facts from one individual to another, e.g. when patients tell nurses that they are in pain or when a radiographer shows a patient how they need to position themselves for an X-ray

● **Supportive communication** – to provide understanding, sympathy or encouragement to patients, e.g. in the face of terminal diagnoses, unpleasant treatment or bereavement.

Hall *et al.* (1988) identified these two key goals in a medical encounter, describing them as 'instrumental tasks' (e.g. asking and answering questions) and 'socio-emotional tasks' (e.g. social conversation and partnership building). As we will see in the next section, factors such as the time pressures under which health care staff work and a clinician's gender result in much communication in health care falling into the former category, despite there being good evidence that the role of supportive communication is both important and neglected. Radley (1994), for example, suggests that the effective use of communication can be therapeutic in itself.

media watch

Patients Reunited

You've bored everyone at work with the saga of your illness. Your partner groans when you mention it. Even your best friends have stopped asking how you are in case you tell them. Where do you turn next?

A new website could be just what the doctor ordered.

At www.patienttalk.com fellow sufferers can chat to each other on message boards exchanging experiences, comparing treatments and providing support.

It sounds like a hypochondriac's dream. But the site's founders say it has a serious purpose.

Penny Stevenson, a former NHS manager and auxiliary nurse, has never run a website before, but she says that patientTalk will succeed because it's putting patients' wishes into practice.

'Patients and their carers have been telling me for years that they need help and support', she says. 'They want to talk about their experiences with someone who's been through the same things.'

Penny is well aware that there are already many support groups doing a great job with few resources. but she believes her site offers something different.

'Support groups for a particular condition are fantastic,' she says, 'but sometimes people will want to speak to patients with other diseases.

'When I worked in cancer services, I met a man with testicular cancer – his testes had been removed. I put him in touch with a woman who'd had a double mastectomy. They were both young and had both lost part of their sexuality. It helped them to talk. You can also remain anonymous on the Internet. Many people don't want face-to-face contact.'

But others are cautious about the need for sites like patientTalk.

'The NHS might not provide all the support that people want, but charities certainly do,' says Simon Williams, director of policy at the Patients Association.

Williams believe patients could be misinformed if there is no medical expert on hand to give advice on a website.

'It's great if patients can learn from each other, but there is a need to treat this source of information with some degree of caution,' he says.

Dr Simon Fradd, who is chairman of the Doctor Patient Partnership, accepts the Internet is giving more people access to health information.

He says: 'Some excellent sources of information can be found on the web that can help people to feel in complete control of their health and more equipped to make health decisions.

continued

'For health professionals, on-line information can often support what goes on in the consultation. For example, if a patient wants to find out more information about a condition or to contact support groups, the Internet is a good starting point.

'Likewise for patients. They may want to prepare for their consultation by looking on-line – this is a good way of maximising on their appointment time. However, this doesn't mean going in armed with reams of Internet print-outs – a balance must be struck.'

And he warns: 'Many sites don't contain the quality information that you would expect from a health provider. People need to be aware of this and stick to well-known, reputable organisations whose sites contain expert and monitored health information such as NHS Direct online and Discovery Health.'

However, Penny Stevenson says that patientTalk will ease the burden on an under-funded and over-worked health service.

'Consultants I've worked with say it's a great idea,' she says. 'They're hoping it will make their job easier by filling a gap that the NHS fails to fill.'

Lucy Jolin from *Take a Break* (2003) 43, 24–25, 9 October 2003.

Reflective activity

The role played by supportive communication can be seen in the interest patients demonstrate for opportunities such as the 'Patients Reunited' website. Consider the following issues raised by the article:

- How might the anonymity of the Internet assist communication for some patients?
- For what reasons might the provision of information be important for patients?
- Why should we be cautious about encouraging patients to use websites?

Communication styles

Communication can be understood from a number of different theoretical perspectives. Many of these models were formulated in the context of general practice, so focus on interactions between doctors and patients in short consultations. These models often discriminate between doctor-centred and patient-centred styles of communication (Table 1.2).

A doctor-centred style concentrates on the practitioner asking the patient questions to obtain information about their medical condition and providing them with advice as a result. The 'communication' is two-way but is directed by one of the participants. In contrast, a patient-centred approach aims to ensure that the patient is treated as an individual rather than a commodity. The patient is an active participant in the interaction, asking and answering questions and responding to requests with opinions as well as facts. As a result, patient-centred consultations are, ultimately, more likely to enable the patients to influence the outcome.

Table 1.2 Different communication styles seen in practitioner–patient interactions		
	Doctor-centred	**Patient-centred**
Focus of doctor	His or her own status and control of the situation	To identify the patient's needs and adjust his or her own activities to satisfy both individuals
Actions of doctor	• Gathers information • Asks direct, closed and rhetorical (self-answering) questions • Asks about medical 'facts' • Decides on outcome for patient and instructs them	• Listens and considers what the patient is saying • Observes and encourages patient to express themselves • Asks about patient's ideas and for clarification, indicates understanding • Involves patient in decision making
Expectations of patient	• Passivity • Ask few questions • Not influence the consultation	• Active engagement • Ask questions • Influence the consultation

Based on Edelmann (2000)

Illustrative of the doctor-centred style, Beckman and Frankel (1984) found that, in the first 90 seconds of a consultation, only 23% of patients were able to complete their answer to the doctor's opening question without interruption, with 69% being cut short within 15 seconds. Similarly, Berry *et al.* (2003) found that, in 55% of consultations with cancer patients, clinicians interrupted when the patient was trying to provide information or ask a question.

Savage and Armstrong (1990) found that patients preferred a doctor-centred consulting style. However, the patients selected for the study were chosen by the doctors as those whom they felt would not be upset by the investigation. This process may, unintentionally, have biased the sample towards those individuals who were more likely to prefer a directive approach.

A patient-centred style of consultation has the advantages of allowing patients to ask questions and providing them with a range of information. This empowerment is preferable for patients – for example, Guadagnoli and Ward (1998) found that patients wanted to be told about alternative treatments when effective options existed.

It might be assumed that all patients would rather communicate in a consultative way but this is not so. Some patients, especially those who are under great stress, including some very ill patients and older adults, prefer the confident, directive style of doctor-led encounters. Others may not want to be involved in decision-making. For example, Blanchard *et al.* (1988) found that, although most wanted information, only two-thirds of cancer patients wished to participate in decisions about their own treatment. Here, the reassurance offered by the absolute opinions of professionals may be more important than the need to feel involved. More recently, Sanders and Skevington (2003) have found that bowel cancer patients similarly prefer to play a limited role in decision-making, so that the responsibility lies with their oncologist. However, Sanders and Skevington also found that these individuals would intervene if they felt that a recommendation was not provided.

Health professionals as skilled communicators

The term 'bedside manner' and its positive or negative connotations suggest that there are good and not-so-good ways for health professionals and patients to communicate. Why is it important that health professionals are skilled communicators? In their interactions with patients, health professionals find themselves dealing with people in personal and physical circumstances that can interfere with effective communication. Patients may be:

- In unfamiliar surroundings
- Interacting with people they do not know well, if at all
- Nervous or anxious
- Embarrassed
- In pain
- Very tired or under the influence of sedative drugs
- Unable to comprehend events, concepts or words that are used
- Unwilling to ask questions.

All these factors are barriers to communication; they will tend to make effective interaction harder. For example, if patients are reluctant to ask questions, this makes the task of judging whether they understand more difficult. However, good patient care relies on an effective relationship between the patient and those working with them. Health professionals need information from patients in order to perform their jobs effectively and ethically, to ensure rapid recovery, and to maximise the patient's comfort and dignity. In this section we will be looking at the skills that health professionals need to employ for successful interactions in even the most difficult situations.

In recognition of the importance of the need for effective communication, the Royal College of Surgeons of England (RCS) has initiatives that aim to provide communication skills training at a range of levels (for senior house officers, consultants, etc.) and place requirements on clinicians to take such training. Membership of the RCS requires new candidates to pass three tests in communication skills and all surgeons are expected to follow the clinical guidelines for communication.

Communication guidelines from the Royal College of Surgeons

All surgeons should:

- listen to and respect the views of patients and their supporters
- listen to and respect the views of other members of the team involved in the patient's care
- recognise and respect the varying needs of patients for information and explanation
- insist that time is available for detailed explanation of the clinical problem and treatment options
- encourage patients to discuss the proposed treatment with their supporter
- fully inform the patient and their supporter of progress during treatment
- explain any complications of treatment as they occur and explain the possible solution
- act immediately when patients have suffered harm and apologise when appropriate.

Copyright © The Royal College of Surgeons of England. Reproduced with permission. The full text of this document can be found at www.rcseng.ag.uk/services/publications/publications/pdf/gsp2002.pdf

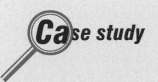
Case study

Kate's communication success

A student health care assistant reported to me an incident that she felt altered her understanding of the importance of communication. An older adult with both physical needs and a severe speech impairment had been given her dinner. She was making a lot of noise – indistinguishable shouts and banging her plate. Her efforts failed to elicit the response she seemed to want. Kate could see the mounting distress on the woman's face and went to sit with her. The woman began picking up her food with her fingers and turning to look at Kate. Continuing to ask her what was wrong, Kate waited. The woman maintained eye contact, as if asking for something, but couldn't achieve an intelligible answer. Instead, she continued to pick at her food, grasping chips between her fingers and banging them up and down on the plate. In a sudden moment of inspiration, Kate took a guess that this might be a gesture, stood up and told the woman she would be coming back. When Kate returned, the patient had maintained the cacophony but, when Kate sat down and the patient became aware that Kate was clutching sachets of tomato ketchup she fell silent and smiled, then cried. She had simply been unable to communicate a basic desire. Kate had been patient and watchful and had, as a consequence, improved her patient's quality of life.

Reflective activity

Re-read the case above and identify the following:
- Examples of good communication skills
- Barriers to communication
- Non-verbal aspects of communication.

Spoken communication

Speech

'Spoken communication' is used exclusively to refer to actual speech whereas 'verbal communication' can be used to mean any word-based communication, so also includes written messages, **fingerspelling** (see page 41) and words depicted in **Braille**. Speech is an enormously flexible and expressive medium. It enables us to communicate any information or feeling for which we can find words. There are few instances in which we find ourselves 'lost for words', although you are likely to be confronted with these occasionally in health care settings.

Reflective activity

Emotions – for example fear, rage, misery, disbelief or being overwhelmed (with relief or pain) – may affect our ability to communicate. These states can be triggered by our own ill health, bereavement, our feelings for sick loved ones or our experiences with colleagues. The environment, such as being in an entirely unfamiliar situation, may also affect us, making us less competent communicators.

Think of instances in which you, a patient, a colleague or a visitor has been 'lost for words'. Under what circumstances did this arise? What reasons do you think might account for your examples? In these situations, what other cues tell us what a person means or how they feel?

Keywords

Jargon
Inappropriate use of professional terminology that excludes individuals, such as the patient or their supporters, from the interaction

As in any profession, health care relies on a vast vocabulary of specialist terminology. You are probably wrestling with learning new terms and concepts at the moment and will become fluent in the 'register' or language of health care. Patients are disadvantaged by being unfamiliar with the terms and shorthand that health care professionals use in their day-to-day speech. When the register is misused, excluding the patient from the interaction, it is referred to as **jargon**. Hadlow and Pitts (1991) investigated people's knowledge of common medical terms and found that doctors understood 70% but patients understood only 36%. Furthermore, according to Roter and Hall (1992), patients are reluctant to ask for clarification if they do not understand. Patients may find their lack of understanding frightening or isolating, may feel that staff are deliberately excluding them or may be angry with themselves. However, sometimes the health care register, acting as a 'badge' to indicate status, may provide a cue that reassures patients that they are in safe hands. In contrast, some patients will be well versed in the current terminology and feel insulted if medical staff 'dumb-down' their explanations.

McKinlay (1975) investigated the extent of patients' knowledge of technical terminology by recording the words used by doctors to, or in front of, patients on a maternity ward. He tested the patients' actual understanding of the most commonly used terms and compared this to the knowledge attributed to them by the doctors. The patients' knowledge was in fact quite high and, importantly, much better than the doctors had assumed. Guidance aimed at surgeons suggests that they should 'recognise and respect the varying needs of patients for information and explanation' (Royal College of Surgeons 2003). This serves to encourage effective communication with patients who have a range of existing knowledge and differing needs in terms of desire to understand.

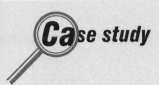

An inappropriate level of communication

A patient who was a well-qualified biologist and health care tutor at degree level reported her feelings following consultations in preparation for a laparoscopy and subsequent hysterectomy. After descriptions of 'periscopes in her tummy' once she had been 'popped under' and 'being pulled together like a draw-string bag' the consultant gynaecologist had failed to inform or reassure her at all. After giving her the opportunity to ask questions, the level of his explanations didn't change despite the patient's obvious knowledge.

Reflective activity

What was the consultant attempting to do? Was he successful? What could he have done to improve his communication?

Jargon may also be used unnecessarily by health practitioners in order to demonstrate their authority, to impress patients or to stop patients asking questions (DiMatteo and DiNicola 1982, Hinkley *et al.* 1990). Both accidental and deliberate use of jargon is detrimental to successful communication. In recognition of this, the World Health Organization (1993) recommended that, in consultations with patients, doctors should:

- Be aware of their use of jargon and consider the patient's need to understand the diagnosis or management of their condition
- Monitor their use of potentially alarming words such as 'cancer' even when used with the intention of allaying fears (such as 'we can be sure it is not cancer')
- Indicate their level of certainty, e.g. in a diagnosis, so that the patient is neither convinced when this is unjustified or left wondering when there is no doubt.

Some benefits for patients have been identified when doctors use 'medical' labels rather than 'lay' labels. In an experimental study, Ogden *et al.* (2003) showed that patients found that a medical diagnosis for stomach and throat problems enabled them to validate their sick role and improved their confidence in the doctor.

Over to you

As you are in training as a health professional, many of the terms that baffle patients will now be familiar to you. To enable you to imagine what it might be for patients, consider how you would feel if you were told any of the following about a problem with your house:

'The A test was negative.' (Is that good or bad?)

'The B are only creeping.' (Should they be?)

'We can detect some C but it's nothing to worry about.' (Isn't it?)

Would you feel safe?

Another problem with the diversity and expressiveness of language is that it can consequently be ambiguous, that is, have two alternative meanings. This can potentially lead to confusion, for example, how should a patient waiting to be discharged interpret the comment 'You'll need to stay in'? In where? Indoors once they get home or in hospital? Another example involved a deaf patient who could use sign language but did not have an interpreter and didn't understand the written question 'Are you opening your bowels regularly?' He definitely hadn't opened anything so replied 'No' and was given daily doses of (quite unnecessary) laxative until he complained of diarrhoea.

Questions

In order to elicit vital information from patients, health care staff need to ask questions. As we have already seen, spoken language is fallible so health care professionals need to take care that they are using questions effectively in order to obtain honest, accurate and complete information from patients and that, in doing so, they are not causing the patient to become distressed. Depending on the nature of the information required, different questioning techniques are used.

Over to you

Barriers to communication

You will need a partner for this exercise and two chairs arranged back-to-back. Do not show your partner the shapes above before you start. Give them a sheet of paper and a pencil or pen and ask them to draw the shape you are going to describe. Warn them that they cannot turn around or ask questions, although they can say 'I don't understand'. Start with either figure, describing the layout so that your partner can draw it. When you think they have finished, both look at the original (keeping the second image covered up). Repeat the exercise with the other set of shapes, this time allowing them to ask any questions they like.

How did the second drawing compare to the first? Why?

What did it feel like to be the one trying to impart information?

What did it feel like to be the one trying to receive information?

What implications do you think this demonstration has for patients and professionals in health care settings?

🗝 Keywords

Closed question

One to which there are only a few possible answers

🗝 Keywords

Open question

One that allows the patient to express him/herself freely, providing longer, detailed answers

---

Closed questions are those to which there is only a restricted range of possible answers. They may be spoken questions, to which the patient can give a limited number of possible replies, such as 'What is your name?' or 'Have you taken this medication before?'. Closed questions may also be used on printed material, such as registration forms, asking 'What is your date of birth' or 'Do you smoke?'. On such a questionnaire, patients may be required to select the most appropriate answer from a list provided (e.g. 'Do you take you take exercise? No/occasionally/weekly/daily').

An **open question** allows the patient to express himself or herself more freely, providing longer, detailed answers. This style of question is an important way to elicit information about a patient's emotions, for example how they feel about their diagnosis or a forthcoming operation. In addition, effectively used open questions may elicit important but unpredictable information that may not be accessible in any other way. This supplementary information may help staff to understand patients' needs more fully. Compare these two short conversations, the first using closed questions, the second open ones. Which leads to better care for the patient?

(A) **Nurse**: Hello, Mr Brown. Are you feeling better today?

Mr Brown: Yes, a bit.

Nurse: I'd like to take your drip out, are you ready for me to do it now you've finished your tea?

Mr Brown: Yes, OK.

(B) **Nurse**: Hello, Mr Brown. How are you feeling today?

Mr Brown: A bit queasy, I think I drank my tea too quickly.

Nurse: Your drip needs to come out, how do you feel about me doing it now?

Mr Brown: I'd rather you didn't – could you do it in a few minutes when I've settled down again?

Berry *et al.* (2003) found that, in consultation with cancer patients, approximately 85% of questions were closed and only 15% were open questions.

Professionally speaking . . .

Asking the right questions

Senior Nurse Advisor
NHS Direct

What kinds of question do you have to deal with most often?
The most frequent calls tend to come from parents regarding children's illnesses, e.g. fevers, vomiting, diarrhoea, rashes and feeding problems.

What are the most difficult enquiries that you have to cope with?
Complex mental health calls can be difficult to deal with.

What additional difficulties do you experience because you are dealing with people on the telephone rather than face-to-face?
The main disadvantage is that you cannot undertake a visual assessment of the caller presenting with symptoms. This is particularly difficult in children as mums are often distressed and concerned, also in the elderly where there can be a tendency to 'play down' symptoms as they do not wish to trouble anyone; you are totally reliant on picking up verbal cues and using questioning skills to gain maximum, accurate information to enable a safe and effective assessment and appropriate onward referral or advice on how to manage symptoms at home. Language barriers can arise, but with the aid of Language Line (interpreter service) we are able to communicate effectively with callers in their own language, so alleviating any additional stress or fears this may cause.

What training or experiences have you had that have helped you to succeed as an NHS Direct nurse?
A varied nursing background, information technology and computer skills, ability to multitask, excellent listening skills, critical thinking, ability to 'visualise' the caller, life experience, empathy and professionalism.

○━♀ Keywords

Leading question
One in which information is
presented that implies that a
particular answer is required
or expected

The wording of a **leading question** implies a particular answer is required. Such questions therefore tend to result in misinformation from the patient and can also cause changes in their memory of what was said. Leading questions may directly or indirectly suggest the possible answer. For example, a woman who is asked 'Would your preference be for a vaginal or abdominal hysterectomy?' would be contradicting the questioner if she volunteered the reply that she did not want a hysterectomy at all.

Consider the following line of questioning:

Surgeon: The operation went very well, are you gaining more feeling in your foot now?

Patient: Yes, a little.

Surgeon: Good, so we'll start you on physiotherapy tomorrow and we'll have you up and walking and ready to return home in no time. That'll be good, you're looking forward to getting back aren't you?

Patient: Yes.

Compare the above to this, alternative conversation:

Surgeon: Are you aware of any change in the amount you can feel in your foot yet?

Patient: Yes, I think there's a little more feeling.

Surgeon: Good, so we'll start you on physiotherapy tomorrow and we'll have you up and walking and ready to return home in no time. How do you feel about going home?

Patient: I'm keen to get home but worried about managing the stairs as I still can't bend my ankle very well.

Which conversation has provided more information about the patient's feelings and physical progress?

Group processes

The spoken language and verbal strategies used in one-to-one situations differ from those used in group settings. Since health care professionals may find themselves working with client groups such as patients and their families, or with a team of colleagues, e.g. at handovers, the differences are important.

Bales (1970) used laboratory studies to determine the patterns of communication used in groups. Some of these are summarised in Table 1.3. These communication strategies may be both causes of and solutions to some of the difficulties experienced in group interactions, such as competition and the need for compromise.

Table 1.3 Patterns of communication used in groups

Group role	Communication function
Proposing	Providing new suggestions, ideas or plans of actions. Generally positive and constructive
Building	Developing or extending other group members' ideas. Also positive and constructive
Supporting	Offering active support and agreement, encouraging co-operation
Dominating	Use of power by an individual or subgroup to monopolise communication
Disagreeing	Indicating disapproval or a difference of opinion regarding the behaviour or ideas of another group member. May be positive or negative
Defensive	Usually preservation of one's own position against attack, disagreement or questioning from others
Attacking	Challenging the contribution or behaviour of other group members, which may provoke defence
Blocking	Using communication to obstruct the proposals or contributions of others. Generally negative
Summarising	Supporting and maintaining the group's work by briefly restating recent or previous contributions
Information-seeking	Eliciting ideas and factual information, or clarification, from others
Information-giving	Contributing ideas, facts and clarification to the group
Inclusive	Encouraging interaction by actively involving group members, especially if isolated or less powerful, for example by seeking contributions from them
Exclusive	Hindering interaction by acting to block the contribution of group members

Listening

When we think of verbal communication our focus tends to fall on the role of speech but, without corresponding listening, spoken words alone cannot complete the communication cycle as any 'feedback' would be unrelated to the initial message. It is common for speakers to use the time when they are not talking to decide what to say next. If this is the case, they cannot be concentrating on listening to the reply. In order to become an effective listener, we need to pay attention to three aspects of the sender's message:

- **Linguistic elements** – the semantics or meaning of the spoken words
- **Paralinguistic elements** – the non-semantic aspects of speech, such as the pitch and volume of the voice, a person's accent, the pace at which they are talking and whether their speech is fluid

or stilted; these can indicate the individual's emotional state or attitude

- **Non-verbal elements of communication** – these are the messages conveyed with a person's body that we do not 'listen to' but attend to through other senses such as vision and touch (see pages 22–28).

Effective listening is an important skill in counselling and, correspondingly, is important for health professionals. Egan (1986) whose counselling model requires effective listening, proposed the following guide to recognising and improving your own communication:

- Face one another **S**quarely
- Have an **O**pen posture
- **L**ean slightly towards the other person
- Maintain good **E**ye contact
- Try to **R**elax but pay attention.

The acronym SOLER may help you to recall these ideas but, remember, they are only guidelines not inflexible rules. A very open posture may suggest to a patient that you are not sufficiently professional, which may reduce the effectiveness of communication. Similarly, in discussion about symptoms or treatments that are very personal, patients may be too embarrassed to discuss them while looking you in the eye.

Over to you

Identify whether each of the following messages that might be attended to by a listener are linguistic, paralinguistic or non-verbal:

- A patient who is talking loudly and quickly, indicating that they are angry
- A visitor who is sitting beside a patient's bed with their arms folded and legs tucked in, looking very white, and who seems to be upset
- A colleague whose speech is punctuated with pauses suggesting that they are anxious
- A hospital receptionist who says that she has booked an appointment for a patient

---

Another concept from counselling is active listening: a way to encourage the client to explore their thoughts and feelings. Active listening can use the following techniques:

- **Mirroring** – reflecting back the client's words or postures to encourage expansion, e.g. to a client who says 'I feel rather empty', you might reply, 'Empty?'

- **Empathy-building statements** – indicating attention and an attempt to understand, e.g. 'I imagine that . . . .'
- **Silence** – to allow the client uninterrupted time to think.

Care must be taken to ensure that mirroring, whether verbal or postural, is not too overt, as the client may perceive this to be sarcastic, and that re-phrasing of the client's statements gives an accurate representation of their feelings. This can be verified with simple questions such as 'It seems as though you are . . . is that right?'.

Non-verbal communication

The non-verbal aspects of communication provide a context within which spoken messages can be correctly interpreted. These additional cues can subtly alter the meaning of the speech that they accompany.

Paralanguage: the non-verbal aspects of speech

Paralanguage encompasses all the ways that the voice is used to convey meaning, excluding the meaning of the words themselves. Try listening to some speech – a live show or an interview on the radio, for example. This task is even better if you can tune into a foreign language station. Even though you may have little idea of the content you will be able to identify some aspects of the way the speaker uses their voice. Paralinguistic features that you may be able to identify include:

- **Speed of speech** – is the pace fast or slow?
- **Tone of voice** – high- or low-pitched?
- **Flow** – is the speech flowing or stilted?
- **Volume** – is the speaker speaking quietly or loudly?
- **Intonation** – is their speech animated or flat?
- **Clarity** – are the words clear or mumbled?
- **Fitted pauses** – are they using 'ums', 'ers', grunts and gasps?
- **Silence** – is there a torrent of words or are there prolonged gaps between comments?

A negative tone of voice can have detrimental effects. Milot and Rosental (1967) investigated the effect of the doctor's voice on a patient's willingness to be treated for alcoholism. A doctor with an angry voice was less successful in persuading the patient to undergo treatment. Voice can also have positive effects. Huntingdon

(1987) found that patients were more likely to ask questions, engage in discussion, trust their doctor's diagnosis and follow instructions about treatment if the doctor had a warm, friendly tone.

> ### ✍ *Over to you*
>
> On page 16 we talked about ambiguity in spoken language. Our use of tone can introduce further meanings to the same words. Working in pairs if possible, try repeating these phrases in as many different ways as you can – what different understandings do you gain from identical words simply because they are said differently?
>
> - 'You can do that'
> - 'Why won't you take these?'
> - 'How did you end up like that?'
> - 'We will come and do it later'
>
> When you've tried these out, consider how many of the adjectives in the box (left) would describe the kinds of expression that you used.

- Pleading
- Instructional
- Encouraging
- Annoyed
- Questioning
- Confident
- Positive

Facial expression

Our faces are very expressive. In addition to obvious cues such as tears, we can begin to judge a person's emotional state from their face. Our facial muscles enable us to move our mouths, eyes, eyebrows and foreheads, both voluntarily and involuntarily, giving others an indication of how we feel.

According to research conducted by Matsumoto and Ekman (1989), the production and interpretation of facial expressions, at least the most frequent ones, is very similar for people of different cultural backgrounds – anywhere in the world, smiling means that a person is happy. These expressions seem to be spontaneous rather than acquired. People who have been blind from birth, so cannot have learned their facial expressions by copying others, display the same facial expressions for these basic emotions as sighted people (Galati *et al.* 1997).

Our facial expressions are important for others to understand us. When they are absent, such as in telephone calls or e-mails, we find judging someone's emotional state much more difficult. In social text, such as e-mail or mobile phone text messages this is sometimes overcome by the use of 'emoticons' such as ;-) for a wink and :-(for a frown – they help to avoid misunderstandings.

Gaze

Eye contact between communicators is an indicator that they are paying attention; it can also indicate expectation, concern or sincerity. Prolonged eye contact, however, is threatening.

Gaze also helps us to take turns effectively in conversation. We tend to look directly at the other person when we have finished speaking, indicating that they may begin. If we simply pause and intend to continue, we tend to look down. Eye contact is thus an indicator that we are about to stop (or start) speaking. This regulates the 'turn-taking' aspect of effective communication. When it breaks down – for example over the telephone or if somebody persistently interrupts – communication is less effective.

Unlike facial expressions, the role of eye contact in communication is culturally dependent. The use of eye contact to regulate turn-taking is typical of British and American spoken language. By convention, in some cultures women do not make eye contact with men except in intimate situations; in others, social status dictates whether eye contact is appropriate.

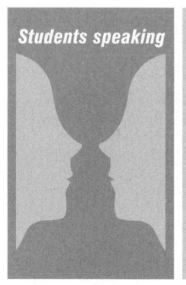

Students speaking

Talking about talking

Second year student nurse

Q: When you talk to patients, do you think it is important that they can see your face?
A: I think it's really important.

Q: Why?
A: Because I always think you can tell a lot from facial expressions, like whether patients are in pain. It's also polite to look people in the face.

Q: What do you do to try to ensure that they can see you easily?
A: Sometimes I crouch down to the person's level, if they are sat in a chair.

Q: Do you think that you ever have to try to mask your facial expressions and if so why might this be important?
A: I have had to do this. Particularly when a patient has a diagnosis of cancer that I know about but they haven't been told of this yet.

Gestures and postures

Gestures are movements; these may be executed with the whole body, as in an exaggerated shudder, or more commonly with the head or arms and hands (such as shrugging, waving and indicating shapes and sizes). Health professionals should be aware that there are cultural differences in the use of gestures and it should not be automatically assumed that a friendly gesture in one culture is equally acceptable to all. For example, 'thumbs up' and waving with the fingers apart, while pleasant signs in Britain, are not regarded as such in all cultures.

> ### Over to you
>
> The next time you are having a day-to-day conversation with a friend or member of your family, try standing back to back with them and let your arms lie by your sides (don't fold them). See how long you can keep going before you try to express yourself using your hands!

Postures are static body positions. Sitting (or standing) up straight or, alternatively, slouching, are two postures that convey opposite messages. A formal, upright posture is assertive, a slumped position more passive. An 'open' posture is one in which the limbs are held relatively far from the body, arms hanging to the sides or stretched out on a table. In a 'closed' posture the limbs are held in, as if to 'protect' the body, for example with the arms folded or legs crossed beneath the body. Open postures indicate confidence; closed postures suggest insecurity. Leaning forwards, towards another person, may also indicate confidence or friendliness but can also be – or appear – aggressive.

> ### Over to you
>
> Record a TV discussion programme and watch it with the sound turned down. Set the timer, if you have one, and use a pre-written sheet with 30-second or 1-minute intervals marked down the margin. Look for examples of non-verbal communication. Try to identify the emotions being expressed and note them alongside the appropriate time. Watch the video again, this time with the sound on, and decide whether you had correctly interpreted the emotions from the non-verbal information alone.

Touch and personal space

We have, around our bodies, an invisible 'bubble', our personal space into which we only tolerate invasion from particular individuals. The more intimate our relationship with the person, the further they may enter into our personal space. Hall has identified four zones based on the distances between individuals with different relationships (Table 1.4). The ranges of these zones vary with culture, some being more tolerant of people standing close to them and of gestures involving touch.

Table 1.4 Personal space zones

Zone	Distance (feet)	Typical relationships and behaviours	Possible sources of communication
Intimate	$0–1\frac{1}{2}$ (0–0.5 m)	Contact is intimate (e.g. between partners having sex, comforting someone with a hug or treating a patient)	Touch is the predominant means of communication, although smell and skin temperature may also be informative
Personal	$1\frac{1}{2}–4$ (0.5–1.2 m)	Contact is close (e.g. between friends, encounters in shops, talking to a patient in a bed or chair on a ward)	Speech is the main communication channel, accompanied by paralinguistic and non-verbal cues. Touch can still be used
Social	4–12 (1.2–3.7 m)	People maintain a distance from each other (e.g. in business situations, small meetings, spoken consultations in an office or across a desk)	Speech is the main communication channel, touch is no longer available but other non-verbal cues can be used
Public	12+ (3.7 m)	Formal settings such as giving a presentation or speaking at a large meeting	Speech, sometimes amplified, is the main communication channel. The greater the distance the less the recipient can gain from non-verbal cues

Over to you

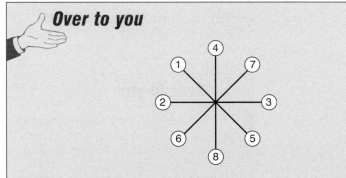

Draw the shape above several times on separate sheets of paper. Imagine you are in the street and standing at the intersection of the lines, facing in the direction of '4'. How close would you allow someone to stand to you before you felt that they were invading your space? Mark across each line in order from one to eight, then join up the marks. Repeat this for several different scenarios – a friend, a stranger, someone you are in awe of. On a separate sheet, consider the same scenario in a health care setting. Imagine you are a patient being approached by a health care professional. Conduct this exercise twice, first picturing yourself as calm and confident and then as if you were nervous. Look at the different shapes that are produced. What implications do such observations have for communication needs in health care procedures that necessarily invade patients' personal space?

This exercise is based on the Comfortable Interpersonal Distance Scale (CIDS; Duke and Nowicki 1972) and is a way to measure the personal space that people expect under different circumstances. The technique allows individuals to demonstrate when an interpersonal distance becomes 'too close' using imaginary situations.

Within a hospital setting, maintaining personal space for patients may be difficult. Conversations that patients may feel should be confined to an intimate zone may be audible to other patients on a ward. Ideally, such conversations would be conducted in a separate room but this may not be practical on a busy ward or safe with patients whose mobility is limited. In order to provide such patients with a greater sense of privacy, curtains may be drawn around the bed. It is worth observing that, for some patients, their own bed is perceived as a 'safe place' and they would prefer to remain there.

When communicating with patients in a confined space, health carers should maintain a distance at which they can be easily heard but are not intimidating to the patient. Remember how invasive you find people standing close to you in a queue or on a bus. Sitting at the same height as the patient helps to avoid the sensation of crowding them and sitting at an angle to them is less confrontational than positioning yourself directly face-to-face.

Touch is a very intimate non-verbal signal often used to indicate affection, for example through hugging, kissing, stroking and tickling. For individuals outside intimate relationships, bodily contact is limited and when it exists – such as in shaking hands – it is highly ritualised. This formality allows a degree of bodily contact that would otherwise be uncomfortable with a stranger. However, health carers need to fulfil a supportive role and this is often enhanced by the use of subtle physical contact. This has to be well judged so as to avoid being invasive but can effectively indicate attention and offer encouragement, or reassurance.

In the process of caring for patients' health there is necessarily a need for bodily contact and health professionals should remain aware that, for each new patient, this has the potential to cause unease. A balance must be struck between formality to help to allow the patient to recognise that the procedure is a necessary part of their care and informality to offer reassurance.

Reflective activity

Think of several examples of instances where you have had to conduct or assist with an intimate procedure with a patient. Such examples might include bathing, toileting or asking personal questions. Describe how you felt and how you believe the patient might have been feeling.

Appearance

Clothing, hairstyle and presentation are aspects of our appearance. Many roles and settings within the health care profession have dress codes or policies relating to standards of appearance. The way a health carer appears can convey several messages.

Most obviously, a uniform indicates role. This is helpful for patients at a practical level – they know who is who – but can also play an important role in reassuring patients who are in a strange environment surrounded by people they may never have met. An individual who is not confident about having a blood sample taken in his local surgery may be reassured by the nurse's uniform. For example, Brosky *et al.* (2003) found that the clothing worn by dental care providers affected the comfort and anxiety experienced by their patients. Conversely, casual clothes may send messages about a lack of care, cleanliness or respect. However, consider what benefits there might be of staff on children's wards wearing less formal clothing.

Health care staff must also be aware that they should not stereotype patients on the basis of their appearance. Jumping to conclusions based on first impressions is discriminatory and will not ensure fair treatment.

Over to you

A health care student was denied a placement because she had three tongue piercings. She challenged the decision on the basis that she had clear plastic retainer studs that were acceptable to her other employer, a supermarket, where she worked on the delicatessen. She was told that they were unhygienic, to which she replied with a letter from her dentist indicating her high level of oral health.

Do you think these steps were appropriate? Imagine the perspective of an elderly patient, a young patient with piercings themselves or a patient with mouth cancer. What decision would you have made?

Factors affecting communication

A wide range of factors has been shown to affect communication. These include:

- **Emotional state** – of all communicators, not just the patient
- **Social and cultural factors** – such as stereotypes, language barriers and the effects of social class
- **Age** – differences in communication and expectations of the young and older adults
- **Gender** – male and female patients, as well as health care workers, differ in communication style
- **Time** – for example to listen to a patient
- **Confidentiality** – the effects of trust and privacy.

Emotions

We saw on page 23 how emotion can be reliably interpreted from facial expressions and how important this is to successful communication – knowing another person's emotional state helps us to correctly interpret the interaction. Some emotions, however, can act as barriers to communication.

Reflective activity

Write a list of health issues that could make patients feel:

- Angry
- Fearful
- Shocked
- Anxious
- Embarrassed
- Guilty
- Isolated

Think of different situations in which you have felt each of the above emotions strongly. Write an account of any problems you experienced when trying to communicate with others on these occasions.

Consider how the effects you may have experienced in other contexts could be suffered by patients undergoing health care.

The emotions of health care professionals are also important. Jeffery (1979) observes that staff may hold negative attitudes towards patients with problems considered to be medically 'trivial', especially when the patients are drunk, homeless or appear to have taken a drug overdose as an attention-seeking behaviour. Such opinions would hinder the ability of the individual to empathise with the patient. According to Rogers (1961), empathy in communication is critical to effective communication. It allows the communicator (the health professional) to understand the perspective of the patient rather than making assumptions about the patient's feelings or what they believe about their condition or treatment.

Social and cultural factors

On pages 23–27 we considered some cultural similarities and differences in relation to the roles of facial expression, gestures and proximity in communication. These are general differences that would relate to many different kinds of interaction.

There are, however, additional cultural differences that relate specifically to health issues, for instance in determining whether an individual perceives symptoms as important, their choice of treatment and whether they seek professional health care at all. In a study of the description of pain by patients, Zborowski (1952) found that Italian Americans tended to complain about their pain in hospital because they could not do this at home, whereas Jewish Americans, who could express themselves at home, chose to talk to the doctor about their concerns about the implications of their pain for their future health. Zola (1966) identified another difference in communication about pain: while Italian Americans reported a wide range of symptoms, Irish Americans described only a few. Similar findings from Lipton and Marbach (1984) suggest that the extent to which ethnic groups have been integrated into North American society affects their reporting of symptoms. One explanation for these differences is the extent to which it is culturally acceptable to express feelings.

The content of messages to patients may also be affected by beliefs about culture. McAvoy and Raza (1988) found that some doctors were not offering contraception to Anglo-Asian women because they believed that it would be culturally unacceptable. Many of the patients, however, were in favour of, and had already been using, contraception. Such errors are based on stereotyped assumptions.

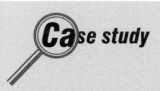

Stereotyped assumptions

A female patient, with long-term dysmenorrhoea, who was on holiday away from her normal surgery was in such pain that she was taken to the local doctor. The GP was helpful and friendly, and was appropriately determining possible causes of the pain, but was misled by stereotyped thinking. Part of the dialogue went as follows:

GP: Could you be pregnant?
Patient: No.
GP: Are you sexually active?
Patient: Yes.
GP: What method of contraception are you using?
Patient: None.
GP: So you could be pregnant then?
Patient: No.
GP: But you are sexually active?
Patient: Yes.
GP: And you haven't been sterilised?
Patient: (*who, by this time, is on the verge of passing out*) No.
GP: So you could be pregnant then?
Patient: No I couldn't – she's my partner (*indicating the person who had brought her to the surgery*).

Think of examples of individuals you know – ex-patients, family or friends – who you feel are counter-stereotypical: people who don't follow generalised predictions based on their age, gender, sexuality, culture or disability, for example. You can probably think of quite a few – suggesting that stereotypes are distinctly unhelpful guides to understanding individuals.

An additional issue to consider in assessing the adequacy of health care provision is whether communication is being conducted in the patient's (or the professional's) first language. Many health services provide printed information in several languages (e.g. in Wales, leaflets are available in English and in Welsh). For face-to-face consultations, however, interpreters may be required if the patient's symptoms are to be correctly understood and they are to receive adequate information about their diagnosis and choice about their care.

Finally, even for patients operating in their first language, there may be differences between sectors of society. People from different social classes tend to report different symptoms and express differing levels of interest in different possible courses of action (Blair 1993). Socioeconomic status is also a determining factor in the effectiveness of health information. Kittel *et al.* (1993) analysed many studies of health communications and found that they were most effective for people of higher socioeconomic status. Janssen *et al.* (1998) found a similar pattern in their investigation of the efficacy of health promotion folders for gay men providing information about the risks of unprotected sex. Their results showed that the materials were only effective for well-educated participants.

One explanation for Janssen *et al.*'s finding is that less educated individuals may not have understood the content. Although now rather dated, one justification for this explanation is that the language used in educational contexts, such as health promotion, tends to use the register of the middle classes. Bernstein (1961) showed that, whilst boys from working-class and middle-class families exhibited little difference in non-verbal performance, the verbal ability of the working-class boys was comparatively low. He suggested that this was because the children used two different 'codes' or languages. The restricted code used by working-class children tended to be less complex, incomplete, reliant on non-linguistic elements (such as facial expression or context) and focused on the present. Middle-class children, in contrast, used an elaborated code, allowing them greater flexibility of expression and understanding as well as the capacity to talk hypothetically. The linguistic possibilities offered by an elaborated code make communications about health matters easier and, perhaps more importantly, health professionals tend to use an elaborated code in their conversations with patients. Individuals who can only operate in a restricted code will therefore be disadvantaged.

Further evidence suggests that patients from lower socioeconomic groups may be disadvantaged with regard to health care. Pendleton and Bochner (1980) observed that patients from higher socioeconomic groups were automatically given more explanation during consultations with doctors and Waitzkin (1985) found that they were offered clearer explanations, reiterating ideas in non-technical terms.

Age

People from different generations have grown up in different social worlds so effectively form separate subcultural groups. In this respect they may have differing beliefs, attitudes and knowledge in relation to health and health care. Of course, many patients will not conform to the stereotypical member of their age-related group and to assume so would be discriminatory. Nevertheless, differences have been identified in the relationships between health care professionals and patients of different ages. Some research suggests that there is a communication advantage for older patients, some that advancing age is a disadvantage. For example, Hooper *et al.* (1982) found that, in interactions with patients aged over 40, doctors spent more time and gave more information than they did with younger patients and, with those over 75, doctors were also more courteous. However, contradictory findings from Greene *et al.* (1986) suggested that doctors tended to pay less attention to psychological issues raised by patients over 65 years old compared to those under 45 and that they were also less patient, engaged and respectful.

As we get older our cognitive abilities change. There are some advantages, such as increased vocabulary and better general communication skills; our memories, however, tend to get worse. Older patients are poorer at recalling information about drug dosage (Kiernan and Issacs 1981) and need shorter, more concise messages if they are to recall effectively (Forshaw 2002).

Effective communication with children may require different skills because, as patients, children are less well able to describe their thoughts and feelings, or do so in ways that differ from adults. Children also differ from adults in their understanding of health and illness. Bibace and Walsh (1979) described the changing conception of health through childhood (Table 1.5). For example, children in the phenomenistic stage may believe that something they did that was naughty caused them to be ill. This may be unintentionally reinforced if they are hospitalised and believe that they have been sent away from their family as a punishment.

Table 1.5 The changing understanding of health and illness through childhood

Stage	Age (years)	Description	Effect on communication
Phenomenistic stage	0–3	The child associates illness with one specific (and often unrelated) 'cause' such as 'Grandma gave me tummy ache' because it happened to start at Grandma's house. They may also focus on one symptom, such as 'Asthma is coughing'	The child may therefore fail to report all the symptoms they are experiencing or ignore the actual cause (if this is unknown to the carers)
Contagion stage	3–7	The child grasps the idea that diseases can be transmitted from one person to another but may over-generalise both the kinds of condition that are infectious (e.g. 'Did you catch your broken arm from your brother?') and the methods of transmission (e.g. believing they can catch measles from a friend over the telephone)	The child may fail to recognise an actual route of infection so will not report it
Contamination stage	7 onwards	The child comprehends the causation of disease by agents such as germs and that these are conveyed by some medium (e.g. the air). They also recognise that diseases may have a range of symptoms	The child's ability to report their bodily sensations and possible causative agents improves
Internalisation stage	7–11	The child begins to grasp the relationship between health (or illness) and behaviour, and that the consequences affect the body on the inside. For example they may describe the effects of cigarette smoke as 'bad for your lungs' or say that eating too many sweets can rot your teeth	The child is more likely to be able to follow health advice as the impact of their actions on their own health is understood
Physiological stage	11 onwards	Factors such as the child's exposure to education increases understanding about body structure, e.g. organs, and both its function and dysfunction. This enables the child to see that there may be many factors that affect health	The child will be increasingly capable of understanding scientific explanations of the cause and effects of their own illnesses or those of others if these are given in terms they are familiar with. Prior to this the child may be unable to understand the purpose of treatments and, when these are unpleasant, may become confused and upset
Psycho-physiological stage	12–14	In this final stage, the child begins to comprehend the role of both physical and psychological factors in health, e.g. that stress can make people physically ill and that being unwell can be a source of stress	Children at this stage will also be able to follow logical, reasoned arguments so will be better able to enter into discussion about alternative treatments

Even though an ill child's understanding of their condition may be different from that of an adult they should still be given information about their illness and treatment. Some evidence suggests that preparing children for their treatment may be counterproductive as it increases fear (e.g. Faust and Melamed 1984). Most research, however, shows that children benefit from being given information about their condition and treatment, such as what procedures will feel like and how long they will last, and having the opportunity to express their feelings and ask questions (e.g. Roberts *et al.* 1981).

The communication of honest information is also important for terminally ill children, who, like terminally ill adults, tend to have a better understanding of the seriousness of their condition than health care professionals believe. Because the death of a child is so traumatic for the adults involved, both staff and parents, the child often receives less information than would an adult in a similar situation (Spinetta 1974). This can lead to a sense of being excluded, preventing the child from expressing their fears or asking questions so they may harbour distressing (and incorrect) beliefs (Bluebond-Langner 1977).

Reflective activity

Communicating with children

The example below illustrates a terminally ill child's comprehension of her own death. How could the situation have been managed differently?

Sally: Peter's bed's empty. Did he die last night?

Doctor: Yes, he did.

Sally: He had the same thing as me, didn't he?

Doctor: Yes, but your treatment is different, so you'll get better.

Sally: Peter's treatment didn't make him better.

Gender

Evidence suggests that health care professionals communicate differently with male and female patients. Some of these differences favour women, others men. Hall *et al.* (1988) found that female patients were more likely to be given information than male patients and this may be in part because they are more likely to ask questions (Waitzkin 1985). Further evidence, from Hooper *et al.* (1982), suggests that female patients not only get more information from their doctors but that this is more comprehensible and that they are less likely to be interrupted and are more likely to get an empathetic response than male patients. In consultations with female patients, doctors also make a greater effort to build a relationship, offer more positive communication, seek opinions and feelings and use 'tension release' such as laughter (Stewart 1984). These differences may, however, arise at least in part because women are more skilled communicators and more willing to express their needs than men so elicit more effective communication from their doctors (Weisman and Teitelbaum 1989).

In spite of their apparently more successful communication, the health concerns of women may be treated less seriously than those of men and are more likely to be attributed to psychosomatic causes. Marshall and Funch (1986) found that men with colorectal cancer were given a definite diagnosis earlier than women and Redman *et al.* (1991) found that, even when objective measures of psychological disturbance were the same for male and female patients, doctors were more likely to see female patients as disturbed. This may account for the tendency to dismiss women's concerns. Oakley (1980) found that doctors argued with pregnant women regarding their due dates – implying that the women lacked knowledge – and were dismissive in their answers to questions about pain and discomfort. Experiences such as this affect the confidence that women have in the health professionals that they encounter.

Communication by female patients may also be hindered by their deferential approach to health care professionals. In a study of economically disadvantaged female patients, Blaxter and Paterson (1982) found that their attitude of gratitude and trust led them to fail to take steps to change their doctor if they felt that their care was not satisfactory, because they did not feel empowered to do so.

Important differences in communication also exist between the ways that male and female medical practitioners conduct their consultations (Martin *et al.* 1988). Female health care professionals are perceived, both by other professionals and by patients, as more willing to listen and more empathetic. Furthermore, patients seen by female doctors are more satisfied with their care. Other studies have found similar results that might help to account for differences in satisfaction, such as West (1984), whose findings suggest that male doctors interrupt their patients more often and use this as a technique to exert control. Roter *et al.* (1991) found that both female doctors and their patients engaged in more discussion, that this was more positive and gave rise more questions and answers than was the case in consultations with male doctors. Such differences in communication may account for the stronger partnership experienced between female doctors and their patients. Many of these differences reflect a general difference in consultation style (see pages 9–11), with female doctors being more patient-centred and male doctors more doctor-centred (Meeuweesen *et al.* 1991).

Time available

Surprisingly, there does not seem to be a direct link between time spent with a patient and either the quality of information exchanged or the patient's satisfaction (Korsch and Negrete 1972). However, as we saw above, there are differences between male-led and female-led consultations and evidence suggests that patients are more satisfied with female doctors. This may in part be because their consultations tend to be longer. Roter *et al.* (1991) investigated the length of consultations and found that, for female patients, consultations with female doctors lasted on average 4 minutes longer than those with male doctors.

Language

As we discussed on page 31 (and page 16 with regard to deaf people), patients or staff who are not speaking in their first language or for whom the use of an 'elaborated code' is unfamiliar may experience communication problems. These difficulties may be exacerbated by the use of technical language or, equally, by efforts to 'simplify' language that introduces inappropriate words such as 'pop into that cubicle and slip this gown on'.

Over to you

Barriers to communication

You may have first hand experience of trying to communicate in a second language, if not, this is a useful exercise to help you to experience what it is like to be unable to find the words to express yourself. You will need to work with a partner.

Write out the alphabet in large letters across the middle of a piece of paper. Fold the paper in half so that you can only see either the first or the last half of alphabet. Using only words that begin with letters in the half of the alphabet you can see, try to tell your partner about yourself, where you live, what you like doing, how you are going to spend your weekend. Swap roles between speaker and listener and use the other half of the alphabet.

How did you get on? Probably, you knew exactly what you want to say; it was 'in your head' but you couldn't find a way to explain it.

Key points **Top tips**

- If you have not yet studied reflective practice, you might find the example described on pages 119–122 of Jasper, *Beginning Reflective Practice* (2003) useful.

Confidentiality

You will have considered the need for confidentiality and the rights of patients in the health care setting. Our interest here is in the role that confidentiality plays in communication. Patients need to know that they can trust their health care professionals not to divulge their personal information to others. This is important to the quality of the communication between the patient and their care staff.

Over to you

Read the following examples and consider how the individual's belief that their confidentiality will be respected would affect communication with the patient or colleague.

- Darren has an appointment with his college nurse for a BCG booster. He's worried about it making him ill as he's recently taken some Ecstasy. He wants to tell the nurse but is scared his teachers will be told.
- Jennifer is having a sexual relationship with her boyfriend and wants to go to her GP for the contraceptive pill. She is only 15.
- Eileen has terminal cancer and is dying. She tells her nurse that she doesn't want to talk to her family but she appears to be very lonely.
- A man with a stab wound arrives at the hospital Accident & Emergency Department. He doesn't want to give his name and asks the nurse not to phone the police. He says he will leave if they do. He is bleeding profusely, is confused but seems to be suggesting that someone else was involved.
- Stan is an agency nurse who often works on a ward with Chris and Sally. Chris mentions to Sally that he's concerned about Stan. He seems to be distracted. Sally happens to know Stan's family and is aware that his mother is very ill. She can't decide what to say to Chris.
- Helen has a verruca on her toe and is really embarrassed about it. She has asked the practice nurse not to tell anyone.
- Greg and Alice have both started working on a high-dependency ward. Greg is upset about the condition of one of the patients and disagrees with the patient's care. He moans to Alice but has asked her not to say anything in case other staff think he is interfering.
- Derek is recuperating in a cottage hospital but has become quiet and withdrawn since moving from the general hospital. One day he says to a health care assistant that he is frightened to ask the nursing staff for anything because they seem to be busy with other patients and that she's not to say anything because he doesn't want to make a fuss.

To protect individuals from vulnerability, four categories of information need to be kept confidential – information about:

- **Identity** – e.g. name, address, marital status
- **Medical history** – e.g. the nature and progression of diseases and treatments
- **Social circumstances** – e.g. family, sexual orientation, housing, employment
- **Psychological factors** – e.g. details of emotional state, stress levels and mental health.

Any placement or employer should make you aware of their code of conduct with regard to ethical issues such as confidentiality. From the perspective of effective communication, confidentiality is important because it provides a level of security without which patients (and staff) may not feel sufficiently confident to express themselves fully. Patients need to feel comfortable that their personal details are not being discussed by staff outside the required domains and that they cannot fall into the wrong hands. The information with which health care professionals are trusted should therefore be treated with respect. Individuals may fear the process and consequences of disclosure; they may feel that they will be judged or discriminated against on the basis of information they have divulged or that, if misused, even simple facts such as their being in hospital could put them at risk from, for instance, burglary.

Enhancing communication

As we have seen so far in this chapter, many factors arising in health care communications may be either advantageous or disadvantageous. For example, questioning style, eye contact, appearance, age and the gender of the doctor and of the patient can affect the outcome of care either positively or negatively. Other factors, such as becoming emotional, invading the patient's personal space and lack of time, tend to be negative in their effect. In this section we will reflect on some of the ways that we can overcome these barriers by managing communication effectively.

> ## *Reflective activity*
>
> ### Good communication
> Think of an instance when you have engaged in or observed an interaction between a patient and a health care professional that demonstrated good communication skills. Briefly describe the scene and comment on what communication skills, such as choice of words, non-verbal cues and appearance helped the communicator to transmit their message effectively. Think about the ways in which the health care professional facilitated communication for the patient: Was there an attempt to put the patient at ease? Did they ask questions? If so were they open or closed? Did they interrupt the patient?

Special needs in communication

The most important thing you need to remember about communicating with people with special communication needs is that all the same rules apply! You will need to make sure that you are aware of the communication cycle:

- Is your message clear enough?
- Is your message being received?
- Are you receiving feedback?

If the answer to any of these questions is 'no', then you need to decide on an appropriate course of action to remedy the situation, bearing in mind that the later stages of the cycle cannot happen without the earlier ones. You will need to consider what you can do, or what resources (human or artificial) might assist you to send the message more effectively, whether the message is being received and what you can do to solve this if it is not – the answer may be very simple, such as gaining the attention of a deaf person who can lip-read before you start to speak. Finally, ask yourself whether there really is no feedback – you may be able to detect a gesture, or a change in expression or in posture that is indicating a reply. You can then build on this to verify the individual's response.

It is worth noting that the obvious special needs that can affect communication, such sensory impairments, are not the only possibilities. People with learning difficulties such as Down's syndrome or autism may find communication difficult, as may people with acquired problems such as the effects of brain injury or Parkinson's disease. The particular requirements for communicating with people with learning difficulties will vary for different individuals. However, it is always important to:

- Speak directly to the person themselves, not their carer
- Express yourself in a clear, simple way without being patronising
- Be prepared to repeat questions and to wait for and listen carefully to the answer.

Over to you

Look back through the entire chapter. Under each of the headings below, make one or two summary points to identify how you could use that factor to improve your communication with patients and colleagues. Remember, your response may depend on the exact context, the individual or their condition so you may need to note alternatives or restrictions – think about the balance between the absence of a factor and using it to excess.

- The communication cycle:
  - Sending the message
  - Receiving the message
  - Feedback
- Formality/informality
- Supportive/informative communication
- Patient/practitioner focus
- Spoken communication:
  - Jargon
  - Ambiguities
  - Questions: open/closed/leading
  - Listening: SOLER/active listening
- Non-verbal communication:
  - Speed/tone/flow/volume/intonation/clarity/silence
  - Facial expression
  - Gestures
  - Postures
  - Touch
  - Personal space
  - Appearance
- Emotion
- Social and cultural factors:
  - Culture
  - Social class
- Age
- Gender (of the patient or other receiver)
- Time
- Language
- Confidentiality

Some impairments to communication can be assisted with human or technological aids. One that you should be aware of is deafness. Many people with hearing impairments can communicate effectively given appropriate opportunities and/or resources. For example, a deaf person who is fluent in sign language does not have a problem with understanding or being the sender or receiver in a communication cycle – provided that they have access to a sign interpreter. People with hearing impairments use a range of strategies to assist their communication. Look at Table 1.6 to see how you can help.

Table 1.6 Communication strategies for people with hearing loss	
Communication strategy	**What can I do?**
Lip-reading	Ensure that you are facing the person, that your face is in good light and that it is not obscured (e.g. by your hands). Don't exaggerate your speech; be prepared to repeat yourself or rephrase your statements.
British Sign Language	Locate a Sign interpreter if one is available. Direct your questions and answers to the person themselves, not the interpreter.
Fingerspelling	Use fingerspelling if necessary but remember that it relies on being able to spell and deaf people may not necessarily be very familiar with written English if their education has been delayed (see also page 13).
Hearing aids	Be aware that a hearing aid may not provide full hearing: a user may be employing other strategies, such as lip reading, and may find hearing when there is background noise, such as on a busy ward, more difficult than in a quiet environment. Do not shout, because this distorts your voice and makes lip reading more difficult.

Speaking to a person with a visual impairment should be no different from speaking to a sighted person – speaking loudly or slowly is unnecessary and inappropriate. However, it is important to ensure that you have been recognised. This may not be possible from your voice alone, so introduce yourself and anyone else who is with you. Also, try to be aware of those aspects of communication that are missing for the person with a visual impairment and try to inform them verbally – for example if you are leaving the room for a while, intend to make physical contact that would be obvious to a sighted person but might otherwise be a shock or are ending the encounter.

Over to you

A deaf person who is a confident lip reader can follow a great deal of what is being said if the speaker's face is in good light, if they are not exaggerating their speech and if the words are familiar. However, some sounds cannot be differentiated from the speaker's lips alone, so the lip reader has to use context to 'fill the gaps'. Try this exercise to allow you to begin to understand the difficulties faced by lip readers.

Work with a partner, one taking the role of the 'speaker' and the other of a lip reader. The 'speaker' must use silent speech, that is, forming the words without using their voice. 'Read' each word in the list 1–10 in turn, then swap roles and use the second half of the list.

1. Slow
2. Go
3. Jeer
4. Sheer
5. Chew
6. Goo
7. Bright
8. Blight
9. Cheap
10. Jeans
11. Sheet
12. Cheat
13. Lip
14. Rip
15. Chum
16. Come
17. Clues
18. Choose
19. Jaw
20. Sure

Evaluating interactions

Evaluating the psychological aspects of a situation is no different from analysing any other and is a key way to improve the effectiveness of your own interactions. If you have used *Beginning Reflective Practice* (Jasper 2003) in this series, you will be familiar with reflecting on your own experiences. Some sections that are particularly useful now include:

- Pages 16–25
- Johns's model (page 84 onwards) and learning journals (page 152 onwards) are two techniques that apply particularly well to evaluating communication
- Chapter 6, 'Ways of reflecting with others' contains some excellent ideas to help you.

Some questions to ask yourself when evaluating communication skills include:

- Was the interaction formal or informal?
- Was the interaction patient-centred or professional-centred?
- Were there many communicators or just two?
- What role was played by different communication skills?
  - Verbal aspects of speech:
    Questions – were open/closed questions used effectively?
    Level/jargon – did the content inform or exclude the patient?
  - Non-verbal aspects of speech: volume, tone, pace – were these used appropriately?
  - Listening skills: active listening, use of mirroring, empathy and silence – were these used sufficiently and sensitively?
  - Other non-verbal communication: facial expressions, eye contact, gestures, postures, touch, appearance – were these appropriate to the context in choice and extent?
  - Physical aspects such as seating, privacy – did the receiver feel secure?
- Were there any barriers to communication?
  - What were they? – consider:
    Leading questions
    Effects of emotions such as fear or embarrassment
    Impairments and special needs
    Invasion of personal space
    Gender
    Age
    Social factors
    Cultural factors
    Time available
    Language or dialect
  - Were any barriers recognised by (all of) the communicators?
  - Was an attempt made to overcome them?
  - How was this attempted?
  - Was the attempt successful?

- If a similar situation arose again, would you act differently?
  - What would you do differently?
  - Why?

The main reason for evaluating communication is in order to improve it, so it is important that, through the reflective process, you recognise what you have gained or learned from different situations.

> ## Over to you
>
> One way to explore the influence of effective and ineffective communication on interactions is to use role play. The following situations could be used to evaluate:
>
> - A nurse with a patient who has been on the same ward for some time
> - A physiotherapist embarking on their first session with a new patient
> - A plaster technician who is trying to gain the co-operation of a patient who is finding the procedure painful
> - A health care assistant being guided by an experienced nurse.

Conclusions

Successful health care, at any level, relies on effective communication between professionals and patients and between health care staff. In this chapter we have considered a range of factors that affect communication. Some, such as the doctor–patient relationship and the use of medical jargon, are specific to health care settings and many others, such as non-verbal communication and personal space, can arise in any encounter. In the health care setting attention to communication is particularly important as patients may, for a variety of reasons, be unable to communicate effectively, yet the need for their understanding and response may be crucial for their wellbeing. In addition, communication plays an important supporting role in recovery.

By exploring the issues raised by different factors in interactions we have considered ways to improve communication where barriers exist. In addition, we have looked at specific ways to enhance communication in instances where barriers are permanent and specific, such as for patients with sensory impairments or learning difficulties.

Reflective activity

Try to recall the details of two difficult but contrasting interactions between patients and health care professionals in which you engaged or that you observed. Choose one that you feel was an example of effectively used communication skills in which barriers were overcome and another that was less successful because communication problems were not resolved. Picture the scenes and consider how the sender and receiver might have felt in each and how, in turn, these feelings would have impacted on the communication itself. If a less experienced student than yourself were going to find him/herself faced with a similar situation in the future, what advice would you give them?

Rapid recap

Check your progress so far by working through each of the following questions.

1. What is the communication cycle?
2. What is meant by 'patient-centred' and 'doctor-centred' approaches to interaction?
3. What does the acronym SOLER stand for?

If you have difficulty with more than one of the questions, read through the section again to refresh your understanding before moving on.

Key references

Other references are in the main reference list at the end of the book.

Edelmann, R.J. (2000) *Psychosocial Aspects of the Health care Process*. Prentice Hall, Harlow, Essex.

Egan, G. (1986) *Exercises in Helping Skills*. Brookes Cole, Monterey, CA.

Forshaw, M. (2002) *Essential Health Psychology*. Arnold, London.

Hinkley, J.J., Craig, H.K. and Anderson, L.A. (1990) Communication characteristics of provider-patient information exchanges. In: *Handbook of Language and Social Psychology* (eds H. Giles and W.P. Robinson). John Wiley, Chichester.

Roter, D., Lipkin, M. and Korsgaard, A. (1991) Sex differences in patients' and physicians' communication during primary care medical visits. *Medical Care*, **29**: 1083–1093.

Savage, R. and Armstrong, D. (1990) Effect of a general practitioner's consulting style on patients' satisfaction: a controlled study. *British Medical Journal*, **301**: 968–970.

Explaining and changing health behaviour

🔑 *Keywords*

Health behaviours
Actions that are beneficial or detrimental to health

Primary prevention
Strategies that avoid risk and promote health in currently healthy individuals

Health promotion
Strategies employed to enhance public health

Many people – patients and health professionals alike – acquire poor **health behaviours**, tending to do things that compromise health. This chapter explores why these behaviours arise and how people can be encouraged and educated to avoid or limit health problems such as stress and drug abuse. The ideal solution is **primary prevention**, ensuring that healthy behaviours prevail over unhealthy ones; for example hygiene and adequate nutrition, and the part social skills can play in reducing health problems.

Health behaviours can be explained in several different ways; the Health Belief Model and the Theory of Planned Behaviour are discussed in detail. Successful health care requires not only an understanding of why people behave in particular – unhealthy – ways, but what can be done to overcome these problems. The theories discussed are considered with respect to their implications for health education. One way in which this knowledge is used is through health education programmes. Examples are used to explore how **health promotion** can be used to raise awareness and change attitudes towards health issues.

Health promotion, health behaviour and health habits

People tend to engage in behaviours that impair their health and fail to commit to activities that could protect or improve their health. Health promotion aims to enable people to gain control of, and therefore enhance, their own health. This may be achieved through lifestyle changes, such as taking exercise, eating a different diet or reducing alcohol consumption and through preventative practices such as breast and testicular self-examination and dental check-ups. Those activities that people do to maintain or improve their health are called health behaviours. People who engage in poor health behaviours not only compromise their health in the short term but

⚿ Keywords

Health habits
Behaviours relating to health that, over time, have become automatic and may be performed without awareness

may develop poor **health habits**, that is, they may acquire firmly established health-related behaviours that are detrimental. We begin to develop health habits at 11 or 12 years old and they may become so automatic that we perform them without awareness.

> **Over to you**
>
> Can you remember cleaning your teeth this morning? It's probably a health habit that is so automatic you don't recall doing it. Now consider your answers to the questions below about the seven health habits studied by Belloc and Breslow (1972):
>
> - How many hours sleep do you get?
> - Do you smoke?
> - How often do you eat breakfast?
> - How many alcoholic drinks do you have on average per day?
> - How often do you exercise?
> - Do you eat between meals?
> - Are you overweight?

Good health habits are important. Belloc and Breslow (1972) asked almost 7000 Californians about the seven health habits listed above. Those who: slept 7–8 hours per night, did not smoke, always ate breakfast, had no more than two alcoholic drinks per day, took regular exercise, did not eat between meals and were not more than 10% overweight had fewer illnesses and were less 'disabled', for instance in terms of days taken off work. When the participants were followed up almost 10 years later, those who engaged in the seven health habits were found to have a lower mortality rate (Breslow and Enstrom 1980).

Primary prevention measures

Positive health behaviours

- Eating a balanced diet
- Eating less fat, salt and cholesterol
- Eating more fruit and vegetables
- Regular dental check-ups
- Self-examination (breast/testicular)
- Taking exercise
- Keeping vaccinations current
- Practising safe sex
- Regular cervical smear test
- Wearing a seat belt

continued

Avoidance of health-compromising behaviours:

- Stopping smoking
- Stopping drug misuse
- Reducing alcohol consumption
- Avoiding stress

Primary prevention

Primary prevention aims to prevent disease in currently healthy individuals by developing good health habits and discouraging poor ones. Two strategies logically follow from this approach to health. First, behaviour change can be used to encourage people to substitute good health behaviours for poor ones, as in programmes to help people to lose weight by altering their eating habits and exercise patterns. Secondly, programmes may aim to discourage people from ever developing poor health habits, for example, educational campaigns to dissuade teenagers from starting smoking or trying drugs. Prevention is clearly preferable but may be difficult to achieve because:

- The range of behaviours known to be threatening to health is limited – for example tobacco, opiates and cocaine have all, historically, been believed to be beneficial to health
- Early intervention may be hindered – even school-based programmes will be too late to protect young people against poor health habits acquired in the home. For example, children of smokers are more likely to smoke than children of non-smokers
- The cognitive limitations of children younger than school-age may prevent full comprehension of the need for health behaviours
- Developing successful strategies to prevent the acquisition of poor health habits depends on understanding this process but our knowledge of the development of such processes is poor
- During the time when people acquire health-compromising behaviours they fail to recognise or accept the long-term threat and therefore lack any incentive to avoid the behaviour.

Hygiene

Historically, greater advances in health have been made through improved understanding of hygiene, that is, avoiding infection through cleanliness, than have been gained through modern medicine.

Helman (1994) suggests several aspects of culture that affect hygiene (either positively or negatively) and therefore affect health. Different cultural practices may:

- Encourage or neglect personal hygiene
- Determine whether, or how often, hair is washed and cut
- Affect choice of clothing – how often it is washed and how tightly it fits (tailored clothing may provide an environment that encourages fleas or lice)
- Dictate the frequency of bathing and whether it is communal or private.

Other hygiene factors that contribute to health include food storage, preparation and cooking; water sources (for drinking and bathing); disposal of human waste; and the location and care of pets and domestic animals (Helman 1994). These issues may be, at least in part, culturally determined.

Further studies have contributed to our understanding of the cognitive and behavioural constraints upon hygiene. Pinfold (1999) used a range of media to convey messages about hand and dish-washing to combat diarrhoeal infections in a population in the Khon Kaen province of Thailand. The use of posters, stickers, leaflets, comic books, songs, T-shirts, badges and a slide show combined to produce an increase in both health behaviours, as indicated by presence of traces of faeces on the fingertips. Schools were more active in the programme than were villages and school children demonstrated a significant increase in knowledge about hygiene. Although knowledge was related to recall of messages contained in the media, this increased knowledge did not necessarily result in improved hygiene-related behaviours. Janis and Feshbach (1953) have also illustrated that information is not the only factor affecting changes in health behaviour (see the summary on page 50).

Janis and Feshbach 1953

Aim: To test whether fear is an effective motive to induce a change in health behaviour.

Procedure: Three 15-minute films were made of illustrated lectures presenting information about the dangers of poor oral hygiene. The recordings differed in their capacity to elicit fear:

- **Strong**: focused on pain (e.g. from tooth decay) and other risks such as blindness and cancer and used photographs of decayed mouths
- **Minimal**: used diagrams and X-rays, avoided serious consequences other than decayed teeth and cavities
- **Moderate**: created an intermediate level of fear.

Each film was shown to a group of students and a fourth group saw no film. Those students who saw the films were asked how they felt immediately afterwards and completed questionnaires about their dental hygiene one week before and one week after viewing the film.

Findings: The strong fear appeal film created the greatest immediate concern and participants expressed greater motivation to look after their teeth. It also aroused the most interest but was rated negatively as it was unpleasant. After one week, however, the high fear arousal group could remember less information and the minimal fear group demonstrated the greatest change in behaviour, with 36% (compared to 8% of the strong fear appeal group) reporting improved oral hygiene habits.

Conclusion: Although fear appeals generate strong emotional responses, these do not necessarily translate into changes in health behaviours such as dental hygiene. The fear elicited by such strong communications does not motivate health behaviour but results in individuals ignoring the problem or minimising the importance of the threat as a result of their fear.

Primary prevention in intravenous drug users

Needle-sharing by intravenous drug users (IVDUs) is a significant risk factor in the transmission of disease because blood remaining in a needle or syringe can be injected directly into another user. Failure to engage in hygienic alternatives (sterilising needles or cleaning them in bleach) results in a high infection rate. It has been estimated that, in Edinburgh, 60% of drug users who inject are human immunodeficiency virus HIV-positive (Plummer 1988).

In addition to AIDS, other diseases, such as hepatitis B and C, can also be transmitted via this route. Whilst it is possible that needle-sharing correlates with other high-risk behaviours, evidence suggests that use of shared IVDU equipment is the major source of infection. Page *et al.* (1990) found that 104 of the 230 IVDUs they studied were HIV-positive. They not only shared needles but also used the same container of water to clean their syringes and prepared injections from shared drug sources, increasing the risk of spreading disease.

In a study conducted by Newmeyer *et al.* (1989) many IVDU participants shared needles and, although they cleaned their equipment, this was in general just rinsing in water. Needle-sharing often arises because needles are in short supply, for example when it is illegal to possess them outside a medical context. Newmeyer *et al.*'s findings suggested that, of possible strategies for reducing infection (including ceasing drug use, injection of drugs or sharing of equipment), only the option of disinfecting shared equipment was acceptable to most IVDUs. Newmeyer *et al.* concluded that, since changing the sexual practices of IVDUs (another high risk factor) would be harder than changing needle use, the latter was a better focus for interventions to improve health-related behaviours.

Junkieboden is a federation of Dutch self-help groups that was involved in the establishment of the first syringe exchange for IVDUs in The Netherlands. Since the needle exchange network was formed, many more individuals have joined treatment schemes, even though the number of IVDUs in Amsterdam has remained constant. The rate of HIV infection has decreased over the same time period (Marks *et al.* 2000). Blakey and Frankland (1995) worked with a target group of prostitutes in Cardiff. The women were provided with information about safer drug use and (in addition to employing safer sex strategies) they reported needle exchange use and reduced needle-sharing.

Several recent studies investigating the use of needle exchange programmes suggest that they make a significant contribution to the reduction of the spread of disease among IVDUs (Vertefeuille *et al.* 2000, Longshore *et al.* 2001, Gibson 2001). Miller *et al.* (2001) interviewed attenders at a syringe exchange programme in Oslo, Norway, between 1992 and 1997, and found that syringe sharing declined significantly over time. HIV prevalence remained low and neither attendance at the syringe exchange programme nor the number of syringes exchanged increased. This suggests that the syringe exchange programme was contributing to the control of disease without increasing drug use. Similarly, Yoast *et al.* (2001) reported on exchange, free distribution and legal pharmacy sales of needles and syringes and found that these neither increased existing drug use nor led to the initiation of drug use.

Nutrition

Health behaviours relating to nutrition most obviously include weight control but also relate to healthy eating in terms of the provision of sufficient and appropriate nutrients. According to Seidell and Rissenen (1998), 14% of the population of England is clinically overweight to the extent that their obesity will adversely affect their long-term health. The additional demands placed on health services resulting from poor nutrition account for the interest governments show in promoting healthy eating habits. Chronically obese people are at greater risk from problems such as heart conditions and diabetes than non-overweight people.

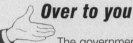

Over to you

The governmental consultation paper 'Our Healthier Nation' states that:

A good diet is an important way of protecting health. The amount of fruit and vegetables people eat is an important influence on health. Unhealthy diets, which tend to include too much sugar, salt and fatty foods, are linked to cancer, heart disease and stroke as well as tooth decay. Research suggests that a third of all cancers are the result of a poor diet.

What health behaviours and health habits do people acquire that perpetuate healthy or unhealthy diets?

In many parts of the world food is in short supply; malnutrition and starvation are appallingly common. In stark contrast, the difficulties for inhabitants of developed countries with regard to nutrition are, most significantly, weight control, although eating disorders and poor diet are also problematic. Humans have evolved to attend to the nutritional needs of active hunter-gatherers so are highly motivated to consume high-calorie, and therefore fattening, foods. As a result people prefer the taste of fatty and sugary foods even though they are probably unnecessary in terms of energy output.

The task for psychology is therefore not simply to understand the desire to overeat but to identify effective ways to control eating. This topic therefore provides us with the opportunity to look at a range of different explanations for health behaviours.

Psychological explanations of health behaviours relating to food

Lay beliefs suggest that there are biologically determined desires for food, as illustrated by the 'food cravings' of premenstrual and pregnant women. Other eating habits are acquired; we might learn not to eat raspberry ice cream because we were once sick after eating some and – rightly or wrongly – formed an association between the two. Finally, beliefs about eating may depend on culture. 'Spinach is good for the blood' and 'Carrots help you to see in the dark' are two such guiding principles (each with a measure of genuine biological foundation). So, health habits such as eating may be governed by three factors:

- Biology
- Learning
- Culture.

To what extent is each of these determinants of our health behaviour important?

Biological explanations

An evolutionary explanation, as proposed at the beginning of this section, can account for the tendency of people to overeat. Not everyone, however, does so. Differences between people may be accounted for by variation in metabolic rate, with obese people tending to have lower rates, utilising energy from food more efficiently and converting surplus intake into fat. Evidence from twin studies suggests that there are inherited components to both basal metabolic rate and the storage of excess energy as fatty rather than lean tissue (Bouchard *et al.* 1990). Such explanations, however, can only account for the way in which excess food is utilised, not the amount that is consumed. This must be controlled by other factors.

Homeostatic theories suggest that our bodies have biological systems that monitor and adjust some aspect of our physiology, such as blood glucose (glycostatic theory), blood fat (lipostatic theory) or weight (set point theory). Each suggests that biological processes, such as hunger, metabolic rate and the laying down of fat, are controlled to maintain the particular variable around an optimum.

In set point theory (Brownwell and Wadden 1992) the hypothalamus (a region of the brain) determines a bodyweight at which an individual will maintain a consistent weight independently of moderate changes in food intake. Each individual's weight is 'set' at a particular point. Thus, according to set point theory, when an individual eats a little more than they need to for weight maintenance, their metabolic rate rises, the energy consumed is used up more quickly and they feel less like eating. Conversely, if they eat too little, the body responds with increased efficiency, lowering the rate at which energy is used and increasing the motivation to eat. As a result, small increases or decreases in food consumption make little difference to long-term weight. This accounts for the failure of crash diets – in the absence of sufficient food, the body may simply conserve energy by lowering the metabolic rate so food is 'burned' more slowly.

Experimental evidence supporting set point theory comes from investigations of extreme eating. Keys *et al.* (1950) observed the effects of systematic starvation. After rapid initial weight loss, the participants' rations had to be reduced to below half their previous intake for them to reach the 25% weight loss target. Re-feeding to return to the previous weight produced a much faster change in weight, suggesting that deviations away from the set point are opposed by bodily processes – the men were hungry and lethargic during starvation but ate up to five meals a day during the re-feeding phase.

In a study into the effects of overeating, prisoners consumed excess food and had restricted physical activity in order to gain approximately 2 stone, or 12.7kg (Sims and Horton 1968). As in the starvation study, initial weight change was rapid but as weight gain slowed the men had to eat around double their normal intake of 3500 calories per day. Some men (even when eating 10 000 calories per day) failed to reach their target, again suggesting that an internal regulatory system maintains the set point. However, in both studies there was a tendency for some individuals to settle above their previous standard weight, suggesting that the internal optimum may be affected by other factors.

Biological determinants of weight, such as metabolic rate and levels of fat cells, may have some genetic contribution. In a study comparing the weight of adopted children to that of their natural and adoptive parents, there was a relationship between the former but not the latter (Stunkard *et al.* 1986). Similarly, identical twins of obese natural parents tend to be obese even when reared apart (Stunkard 1988). Together, these findings imply that inherited factors do play a part in determining weight. They do not, of course, suggest that the environment is unimportant. Indeed, even family trends may be explained by environmental rather than genetic factors. Mason (1970) found that 44% of the dogs owned by obese people were also obese, compared to only 25% of dogs with owners of normal weight.

So genetic factors affect weight, as does energy intake compared to expenditure, i.e. eating and exercise. Since this variable is not inherited, other factors must be considered in the explanation of healthy eating habits.

Behaviourist explanations

Learning theories (see also pages 92–95 and 186) can explain the acquisition of health behaviours. Classical conditioning suggests that we learn associations between a 'new' situation (the neutral stimulus) and an 'old' one (the unconditioned stimulus) to which the individual already exhibits a behaviour (the unconditioned response). Repeated pairings of the neutral stimulus and unconditioned stimulus result in the generation of a behaviour resembling the unconditioned response in response to the neutral stimulus. Once this association has been established, the neutral stimulus is called the conditioned stimulus and the resulting response the conditioned response.

For example, the acquisition of 'comfort eating' may be explained using classical conditioning. Chocolate (unconditioned stimulus) tastes nice so makes us feel good (unconditioned response). In a situation where we are unhappy (neutral stimulus) we can experience an elevation in mood (unconditioned response) by eating chocolate (i.e. pairing the neutral stimulus and unconditioned stimulus), thus we learn to cheer ourselves up with food (conditioned response).

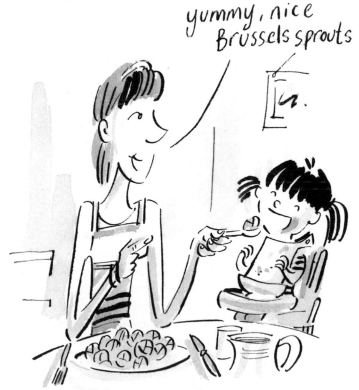

Children acquire good (or bad) health behaviours by imitating the behaviour of adults

In operant conditioning, behaviours that are followed by pleasant consequences (reinforcers) are performed more often, those with unpleasant consequence (punishers) less often. Unhealthy food-related behaviours are often rewarding – chips and chocolate taste nice – thus they are reinforcing and performed more often. Whilst such behaviours do have unpleasant consequences on health (negatively affecting teeth, weight and the heart) their effects are delayed so are ineffective as punishment.

An additional theory, social or observational learning, suggests that behaviours can be acquired by watching and imitating the actions of others. Thus we may like sweets because we see other children enjoying them but dislike vegetables if our siblings protest about eating them. Parents are powerful models for the amount and types of food that children learn to enjoy.

Cultural explanations

Culture can account for some differences in food-related behaviour, including constraints, such as those imposed by Ramadan or Lent, and expectations, such as the consumption of rich foods for celebrations. In addition, cultural preferences may guide choices. For example, traditional foods may continue to predominate in the diet long after international trade has made other foodstuffs readily available.

Over to you

Use the Internet or other resources to investigate food preferences of a range of cultures. In your experience, are such cultural dietary differences considered in the menus offered to patients in hospital? To what extent could this affect recovery? Consider both the physical effects of eating an altered diet and the psychological effects of imposed changes.

Food availability is clearly a factor in healthy eating and, although the presence of excess food will not necessarily result in weight gain, where the abundance includes a variety our choices of food may be unhealthy; fatty and sugary foods taste nicer so are selected in preference. Eating dessert when we are already full depends both on the taste and the social incentive. Variety itself also plays a direct role. Sclafani and Springer (1976) investigated the effect of a wide, variable diet on rats. The experimental animals had free access to 'supermarket foods' including cheese, salami, bananas, chocolate chip cookies, marshmallows and chocolate, and increased in weight by 269%! Since supermarket shopping and access to good storage facilities such as freezers enable people to maintain a huge diversity of foods in their homes, healthy eating behaviours may be compromised by the powerful effect of novelty on satiation. Conversely, this illustrates the importance of offering patients who need to gain weight a varied diet.

Society provides powerful role models, for example within the family and on television. Wadden and Brownwell (1984) found that an average American child watches 10 000 commercials for food every year, for cereals, sweets and biscuits – just 5% were for products that did not contain sugar and none at all were for vegetables. Furthermore, 75% of mothers selected foods chosen by their children, suggesting that advertising directly influences children's diets.

Historically, food has been in short supply, so fatness, rather than thinness, has been culturally endorsed as a sign of health and prosperity. Today, however, developed countries value lower body weights, as illustrated by the declining body weights of Miss America contestants and Playboy centrefolds relative to average weight for the general population (Garner *et al.* 1980, Wiseman *et al.* 1992). These results reflect a cultural preference for thinness but this conflicts with the trend for increasing body weight in society, hence the dissatisfaction of many people with their size. One study reports that two-thirds of the women and more than half of the men questioned were trying to lose, or avoid putting on, weight (Serdula *et al.* 1993).

Key points *Top tips*

Biological
- People are powerfully motivated by the taste of food, especially sweet and fat-rich flavours
- Weight control programmes need to be tailored to individuals to combat the effect of different set points

Behaviourist
- There is a need to counter-condition or unlearn associations that have been built up between unhealthy food and positive emotions or comfort
- Healthy food must be perceived to be as rewarding as unhealthy food
- Reinforcements are less effective if they are not immediate
- Role models must exhibit positive behaviours towards healthy but not unhealthy foods

Cultural
- Children's food choices are affected by advertising and this is not necessarily countered by adults' shopping behaviour
- Cultural differences in eating habits may mean that different health issues arise within different cultural groups

> ### Over to you
>
> Use biological, behaviourist or cultural explanations to account for the following food-related differences in behaviour:
>
> - A child who is bullied in the lunch queue eats the vegetarian option in order to avoid his classmates, although he eats meat at home – later in life he doesn't like eating meat in restaurants
> - Two people of the same height and gender who eat identical diets and take the same exercise are not the same weight
> - Advertisements for chocolate often use images suggesting sex appeal
> - A family that encourages 'finishing everything on your plate' regardless of whether or not you are hungry finds that the children grow into adults who are indiscriminate eaters
> - Parents who tend to overeat have children who also overeat.

Explaining health behaviour

● Keywords

Cognitive
Relating to attention, perception, thinking, reasoning or memory

The health belief model

The health belief model (HBM) is a **cognitive** model that attempts to explain health behaviours by considering the variables that affect an individual's decision making in relation to health-protective and health-compromising behaviours. It was originally proposed by Hochbaum (1958; see box below) and has been adapted several times (e.g. Rosenstock 1966 and Strecher *et al.* 1997).

Hochbaum 1958

Aim: To investigate the factors affecting people's participation in a health screening programme.

Procedure: 1200 adult residents of cities participating in a new tuberculosis screening programme were asked about their beliefs about tuberculosis in relation to themselves and whether or not they had attended screening clinics.

Findings: Two factors were found to predict the likelihood of people participating in the scheme – whether the individual:

- Felt personally at risk of catching tuberculosis
- Believed that early identification and treatment of the disease would be effective.

Of those people who held both these beliefs, 80% went for screening, but only 20% of those who held neither.

Conclusion: Health behaviours are closely related to specific health beliefs. Therefore, a key to effecting change in people's health behaviour is to understand how decisions affecting health are made and thus how the beliefs and consequent behaviour can be altered.

The HBM identifies five core beliefs. These are:

- **Perceived vulnerability** – the individual's assessment of the risk that they will be affected by the condition (i.e. susceptibility)
- **Perceived seriousness** – the individual's assessment of how bad the effect will be if they are affected (i.e. severity).

Together, perceived vulnerability and seriousness determine the individual's perception of the threat posed by the disease. So, for example, a person who is asthmatic may recognise that this is a lethal condition (high perceived seriousness) but believe that because they don't get breathless during exercise they do not need to be concerned (low vulnerability). Where some threat exists, the individual must determine the extent to which engaging in a particular health behaviour will protect them. This is a balance between barriers and benefits.

- **Perceived barriers** – aspects of the situation that disincline the individual to take action. These may be financial (cost of prescriptions), situational (living a long way from a hospital) or social (not wanting to inconvenience other people by being off work). Time, effort and the perception of obstacles would also act as barriers
- **Perceived benefits** – possible gains for the individual (alleviating pain or anxiety, improving health or reducing health risks).

Together, the perceived barriers and benefits present the individual with a cost–benefit analysis. For example, Abraham *et al.* (1992) studied Scottish teenagers, who were well aware of the seriousness of the risk of HIV infection, their vulnerability to it and the benefits gained by using condoms. However, condom use by the participants was prevented because the perceived barrier of costs, including loss of pleasure, awkwardness of use and anticipated conflict with their partner exceeded the perceived benefits of avoiding infection.

- **Cues to action** – for an individual to exhibit a health behaviour, even when the cost–benefit analysis judges it to be necessary, a cue to action is needed, that is, an immediate trigger to initiate the appropriate behaviour. This may be internal or external. For example, a patient may believe that they should stop smoking because it is a serious threat to their health, they recognise their vulnerability and they know that stopping would be advantageous. However, they may only do so on developing severe chest pains (internal cue) or if a relative dies of lung cancer (external cue).

The five core beliefs of the HBM should predict the likelihood that a particular health behaviour will arise in a given situation. Consider an example of a stressed individual with a high cholesterol level who believes that changing their eating habits to reduce their fat intake is going to reduce their risk of dying of a heart attack. They are more likely to persevere with the diet despite disliking it than a person who holds the belief that the fuss about cholesterol levels is all hype (low perceived seriousness) or that no one in their family has heart problems so they are not at risk (low vulnerability).

Over to you

Taking the example of someone who is obese and at risk from heart disease, identify the following statements relating to health beliefs and decide which person would be likely to embark on health-protective behaviours:

Patient A
- 'My chances of having a heart attack are low.'
- 'I don't want to turn into a jogging-junkie.'
- 'Exercising cuts down the risk of a heart attack but even sporty people still have them.'
- 'People who have heart attacks generally recover and go back to work.'

Patient B
- 'Heart attacks kill people.'
- 'I feel ready to start exercising more.'
- 'My neighbour had a heart attack and he was younger than me.'
- 'I guess that being stressed increases my chances of having a heart attack.'
- 'Getting fit will make me more attractive too.'

Evidence indicating that knowledge is important in bringing about appropriate health behaviours suggests that the provision of health information is worthwhile. Rimer *et al.* (1991) found that women who had more knowledge about breast cancer were more likely to have regular mammograms and O'Brien and Lee (1990) demonstrated that manipulating knowledge about Pap tests (for cervical cancer) – by showing women an informational video – resulted in both increased knowledge and healthier behaviour.

However, more information is not always beneficial. The Internet has made an enormous amount of health information available to patients and, despite the popular representation of the Internet as a reliable source of information about health (e.g. Krechowiecka 2001 in the *Guardian* newspaper), much of it is worryingly inaccurate. Matthews *et al.* (2003), in a survey of Internet sites about alternative therapies for cancer, found that, for two of the therapies considered, over 90% of the websites surveyed contained incorrect information. Furthermore, ready access to information about health problems may actually increase anxieties about health rather than providing reassurance.

At least some uses of the Internet are, however, beneficial; Winzelberg *et al.* (2000) successfully used the Internet to deliver a health programme designed to reduce women's dissatisfaction with their body image.

Using the health belief model

The health belief model can be used to interpret behaviour in a number of contexts, for example to understand why people make use of or ignore disease prevention schemes and screening tests. Haefner and Kirscht (1970) found that people were more likely to use disease prevention measures and attend health screening services, including physical examinations and X-rays, if they were exposed to interventions that stressed vulnerability and the effectiveness of the particular health behaviour in combating the risk. Thus, the HBM can not only help us to understand health behaviours but provide a means to improve people's health.

The HBM can, for example, be applied to the situation described by Abraham *et al.* (1992; page 78). The HBM would suggest that an effective AIDS campaign should focus not on vulnerability and seriousness but on overcoming barriers to condom use.

Making use of disease prevention

Schemes for disease prevention include **immunisation**, self-examination (of the breasts or testicles) and effective tooth brushing and flossing. The reason for encouraging people to engage in preventative measures is clear; it reduces health risks and early detection makes treatment easier.

○━┱ *Keywords*

Immunisation
Protection against disease by administering a vaccine to individuals before the infectious agent has been encountered

---

⌐ *Over to you*

Identify how the issues described below would, according to the health belief model, affect a parent's decision-making about whether to have their child immunised.

- **Risk–benefit ratio** – perception that the risks of being immunised outweight the benefits of not contracting the disease
- **Individual risk** – belief that the societal statistics that public health planners use do not apply to their child; further, the parents believe that they can protect the child from exposure
- **Ambiguity aversion** – aversion to options with ambiguous outcomes such that parents will prefer a straightforward Yes/No assessment of the likelihood of their child contracting a disease; when there is a disagreement about potential risk they will err on the side of caution
- **Omission bias** – preference for acts of omission over acts of commission
- **'Free riding'** – assumption that, since most of their children's peers have been vaccinated, they are protected.

From Meszaros *et al.* 1996, p. 698

Immunisation is effective against diseases such as whooping cough (pertussis), measles, mumps and rubella (MMR) and many more. In an interview study of mothers in north-west England, New and Senior (1991) found that fewer than 75% had had their children fully immunised. One reason for not having their child vaccinated against whooping cough was the risk to the child from the pertussis vaccine; in other words, the perceived barriers were too great. Research from both the UK (Reddy 1989) and the US (Lewis *et al.* 1988) has found that parents often fail to take the child for their appointment because they have a minor complaint such as a cold. This suggests that the benefits of vaccination were not perceived to be sufficiently high to overcome other concerns. Lewis *et al.* consider that adverse media reports may have deterred parents from completing their child's vaccination series. Again this suggests that the perceived benefits of vaccination do not outweigh the perceived barriers.

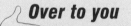

Over to you

Use the Internet to find reports on the public response to MMR vaccination and its potential link to autism. Consider how the health belief model would explain the effect of such publicity on parental choices with regard to immunisation.

Murray and McMillan (1993) investigated the effectiveness of the HBM as a predictor of breast self-examination. A sample of 391 women completed questionnaires about their health behaviours, including the frequency of breast self-examination, and rated items reflecting their health beliefs, such as: 'My chances of getting cancer are great' (susceptibility), 'I am afraid to even think about cancer' (seriousness), 'If cancer is detected early it can be successfully treated' (benefits) and 'I just don't like doctors or hospitals' (barriers). They also provided information relating to their knowledge about cancer, their confidence in performing self-examination and whether any family member had ever had cancer.

The findings showed that breast self-examination was related to many variables, including knowledge and perceived benefits. Demographic variables such as age and social class also affected participation: young professional women were more likely to use breast self-examination. The best predictor of appropriate action in this context was **self-efficacy** – an individual's confidence in their own ability to perform a behaviour. Women who were more confident about carrying out breast self-examination were more

Keywords

Self-efficacy
The extent to which an individual believes they can perform a particular behaviour adequately

likely to do so. This evidence suggests that health promotion should aim to improve women's confidence in their ability to perform self-examination and to provide opportunities to practise the skill.

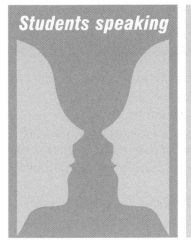

Both anxiety and information are important factors in determining health behaviour

Student nurse in a Day Care Unit

I got some leaflets from the health education centre about testicular self-examination and I asked to put them around the ward. One health carer said that they thought it would frighten the patients, raising their feelings of being at risk. From my learning in college about health belief models I think the availability of leaflets does not necessarily raise anxiety.

Making use of screening tests

Screening tests include cervical smear tests for women, ultrasound scanning, amniocentesis and X-rays. As with disease prevention measures, screening enables health professionals to detect diseases early and treat them more effectively. Participation in these health behaviours can be predicted, and appropriate directions for health promotion ascertained, using the health belief model.

As part of the study described on page 62, Murray and McMillan (1993) investigated the power of the HBM to predict attendance at cervical cancer screening tests. The women were asked how many previous tests they had been for and why (e.g. doctor suggested it or routine postnatal check-up). When compared to measures of health beliefs, it was found that cervical smear testing (like breast self-examination) was related to knowledge and perceived benefits. However, the best predictor was 'barriers'. In other words, the women were more likely to have smear tests if they perceived little threat from the health service, the examination itself or the result. In terms of health promotion this suggests that attendance at cervical smear testing could be improved by education that aimed to reduce the anxiety experienced by women about the consequences of the investigation.

In addition, the benefits of cancer screening are also perceived to be low. Several studies have found that a common reason for non-attendance at cancer screening is that women believe that cervical smear tests are not necessary (e.g. Harlan *et al.* 1991), or only

🔑 *Keywords*

Meta-analysis
A statistical technique that combines the results of many studies

Mammography
X-ray screening to detect breast cancer

important when symptoms were present (e.g. Slenker and Grant 1989). This suggests that perceived vulnerability is also low.

McCaul *et al.* (1996) conducted a **meta-analysis** to investigate factors affecting uptake of **mammography**. There was a strong relationship between family history and attendance, suggesting that perceived vulnerability (as well as actual risk) played an important part in motivating women to attend. Bernstein Hyman *et al.* (1994) found that women who did not attend a scheduled mammogram appointment perceived fewer benefits than those who did. In the absence of a relationship between attendance and perceived vulnerability, they suggested that other factors, such as knowledge, are more important in determining health behaviour with regard to mammography. This implies that more information about the risks of breast cancer and the importance of mammography would improve attendance rates for screening.

Despite the clear evidence for the HBM, there are a number of criticisms. While many health behaviours are affected by the factors proposed, some, such as dieting or exercise, may be motivated by non-health-related reasons, for example a desire to look good. Variables such as this cannot readily be taken into account by the HBM. Another important factor that the HBM, because it is a cognitive model, cannot account for is the influence of emotions. An individual may fail to attend an appointment for a vaccination, even when they hold appropriate beliefs, because they have a phobia about needles – but this emotional component would not be explained by the HBM.

The theory of planned behaviour

Ajzen (1985, 1991) based the theory of planned behaviour (TPB) on an earlier idea, the theory of reasoned action. The TPB proposes that actions, such as health behaviours, are determined by a combination of behavioural intention (deciding to achieve a goal) and perceived behavioural control (believing that you can or cannot perform a behaviour).

So, if we consider the example of someone who wants to give up smoking, the two factors can be distinguished – first, wanting to be a non-smoker (behavioural intention), perhaps to avoid feeling excluded by non-smoking friends, and second, believing that you can achieve the goal (perceived behavioural control), for example feeling that you have the strength to overcome the unpleasant effects of nicotine withdrawal. The importance of both factors is illustrated by the findings of Schifter and Ajzen (1985) in their study of weight loss in female students. Individuals who both expressed the intention to lose weight and perceived that they would be able to

○━┓ Keywords

Attitude

The product of an individual's beliefs in the outcomes of the health behaviour in question and their evaluation of these outcomes

Subjective norms

The individual's beliefs about the value other people (individuals or groups) place on his or her health behaviour and the extent to which there is a motivation to follow these expectations

limit their calorie intake over the 6 weeks of the study lost more weight. This shows that intention only predicts healthy behaviour when perceived behavioural control is high.

Behavioural intention itself may be determined by **attitude** (which is affected in turn by knowledge) and by **subjective norms** arising from our beliefs and inclination to comply with these values. There are two components to subjective norms; normative beliefs about how others expect us to behave and motivation to comply. Considering the smoker again, they may believe that smoking is damaging to the lungs and heart, and may value health and fitness, resulting in an attitude that will make them more likely to give up. In this respect TPB resembles the health belief model as it considers the role of beliefs in affecting behaviour. The smoker may also consider subjective norms such as how their family feels about smoking (normative beliefs) and may be compelled to follow their example or advice (motivation to comply).

The relationship between behavioural intention and action has been supported empirically. Research has successfully applied TPB to a range of health behaviours, including smoking (Norman and Tedeschi 1989), weight loss (Schifter and Ajzen 1985) and breast cancer detection (Montano and Taplin 1991). Eagly and Chaiken (1993) report successful application of the model to other health behaviours such as blood donation, contraception, consumption of junk food, dental hygiene, having an abortion and smoking cannabis.

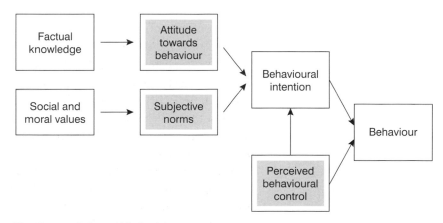

The theory of planned behaviour

Michie *et al.* (1992) found that behavioural intention was a good predictor of the likelihood of pregnant women attending health information classes. Those women who, prior to delivery, expressed an intention to attend classes were more likely to do so once their baby was born. However, factors such as the attitude of the baby's father also contributed to attendance.

Brubaker and Wickersham (1990) investigated the use of testicular self-examination by young men following instruction in the procedure. The participants were also given a questionnaire to establish their attitudes towards this health behaviour, their beliefs about subjective norms, the effectiveness of testicular self-examination as a means of detecting testicular cancer (i.e. outcome), their own effectiveness at testicular self-examination (self-efficacy) and their intention to perform it in the future. When followed up later, the results showed that both attitude towards testicular self-examination and beliefs about subjective norms (such as the extent to which they felt other people wanted them to practise self-examination) significantly predicted intention to perform testicular self-examination.

Povey *et al.* (2000) tested the TPB in the context of dieting. They used questionnaires to measure participants' initial intentions to eat either five portions of fruit and vegetables a day or a low-fat diet and subsequent behaviour (whether the dietary principle was followed). Perceived behavioural control, self-efficacy and beliefs were also tested. These variables were good predictors of intention to eat fruit and vegetables or reduce fat intake, with self-efficacy being a more consistent predictor than perceived control. In addition, attitude related strongly to intention to eat a low-fat diet and subjective norms predicted intention for eating fruit and vegetables. They concluded that self-efficacy was a better predictor of intention than perceived control, which suggests that a person's perception of their ability to engage in a behaviour is an important factor affecting their intention to perform that behaviour. So health promotion strategies that aim to change dietary habits should target people's attitudes and their self-efficacy.

Having the intention to perform a behaviour does not necessarily lead to the behaviour arising. An overweight patient may have decided to diet but may not actually do so. They are more likely to fulfil an intention if it is specific: 'I will not buy chocolate' is more likely to be successful than 'I will eat less'. Latency also affects the link between intention and behaviour. Individuals are more likely to follow an intention through if they perform the behaviour immediately after deciding to do so. Hence, 'I will swim daily, starting today' is more likely to work than saying 'I will start swimming next week'. Thus TPB suggests that advice to patients should be specific and require an immediate change in behaviour.

Being able to predict health behaviour is clearly useful in planning health promotion campaigns, although the effectiveness of any chosen strategy depends on the factors most salient in the decision-making process. For example, in the choice between bottle and breast feeding, women seem to be affected more by attitudes than by subjective norms (Manstead *et al.* 1983). Conversely, a woman's decision to have an abortion seems to be more strongly affected by perceived social pressure (i.e. subjective norms) than by her attitudes (Smetana and Alder 1980).

Such findings have important implications for health promotion. Health behaviours that are strongly affected by the individual's attitudes are more likely to change if the individual is exposed to persuasive information but those behaviours that are primarily the product of subjective norms will be affected by attempts to change beliefs about expectations.

Rutter (2000) used the TPB to predict attendance of women at mammography sessions. A total of 1215 participants who had not been screened before completed questionnaires to indicate attitudes, subjective norms, perceived behavioural control over attendance and intention to attend breast screening. Those women with a strong intention to attend were the most likely to do so, both at their first and their follow-up screening (3 years later). In line with the TPB, their intention was predicted by attitude, subjective norms and perceived behavioural control. The findings suggest that screening rates might be improved in those women who do not attend by focusing on subjective norms – why other people might wish them to attend. Anti-smoking campaigns that feature a child looking beseechingly at a parent and saying 'But I don't want you to die!' illustrate this approach.

Behaviours primarily driven by behavioural intention rather than perceived behavioural control also warrant a different approach to health promotion. Where behavioural intention is not the best predictor of behaviour, this raises the question, why not? The issue here is to ascertain the reasons why behaviour and intention are not related.

Stroebe (2000) suggests that such situations are rare and that, where behaviour is largely the product of perceived behavioural control, there is, in fact, very little variation in intention between individuals. Thus perceived behavioural control becomes a much more potent cause of action. More commonly, behaviour is governed predominantly by behavioural intention so, as well as the factors of attitude and subjective norms that we considered on pages 65–66, the contribution of perceived behavioural control also has to be considered. The case of failed AIDS campaigns provides an appropriate example. De Wit *et al.* (1990) reported a questionnaire study of secondary school children, assessing their health-related

knowledge about AIDS and the following variables in relation
to condoms:

- Attitudes towards their use
- Perceived norms of use
- Perceived behavioural control over use
- Intention to use them.

The test was administered before, and 2 weeks after, the students
saw a health education programme on AIDS. Although this
intervention increased knowledge about AIDS, it did not affect
health behaviour; condom use by the students did not increase.
This was because condom use was governed not by knowledge or
perceived susceptibility but by attitude to condom use and perceived
norms and effectiveness.

These findings have clear implications for improving health
education. More emphasis should be given to changing attitudes to
condom use, subjective norms and individuals' perception of their
own effectiveness.

Changing health behaviours through health education programmes

Health education programmes attempt to change people's health
behaviours from health-compromising to health-enhancing ones.
This may be attempted through different routes according to the
model being followed. For example, fear arousing appeals should,
according to the health belief model, increase perceived vulnerability
– but this approach has little success. Warner (1977) found only
small, transient reductions in smoking (4–5%) following scares in
the USA in the 1950s and 1960s. It could also be argued that a
'shock–horror' approach to discouraging drug use is counterproductive because it emphasise the seductive qualities of any drug.

Kelley (1979) reported on the effectiveness of a mass media
campaign to increase the percentage of car drivers wearing seat belts
(which stood at 6.3% for city driving in 1968). Using cable television
to segregate experimental groups, Kelley ensured that some
households saw professionally made seat belt advertisements
frequently over a 9-month period (estimated at two or three times a
week), while others did not. Using car licence plates to identify
drivers from the two experimental areas, observers counted the
number of drivers wearing seat belts after the experimental period.
The shocking conclusions were that the campaign had had no effect

on seat belt use; drivers from the experimental group did not alter their behaviour at all during the test period. Kelley concluded that mass media campaigns are an ineffective way to attempt to alter health behaviour.

Informational appeals aim to promote good health by providing people with the knowledge to make better health behaviour choices. However, information presented in campaigns may be interpreted differently by the intended recipients from the way it is interpreted by those with a wider perspective. In population terms, nearly 10 000 in every 1 000 000 male smokers aged 35 will die before reaching 45 because of their habit. From the perspective of the individual, however, this is only a 1% chance – the odds are on survival. It is difficult to persuade individuals that they are at risk, so campaigns need to identify and focus on other routes to changing behaviour.

Nevertheless, access to information may still be a barrier. One relatively new source of health information is the Internet. Condon (2001) describes the successful use of Internet chat rooms by the director of San Francisco's Stop AIDS project, Marcel Miranda. The Internet, Miranda suggests, offers a way of getting information about HIV and safe sex to groups who would otherwise remain uninformed.

Over to you

Use your library or an Internet-based search to locate articles about Rachel Whitear, who, it was believed, died from a heroin overdose in 2002. Much was written about her death and a video was produced, aiming to discourage young people from taking drugs. However, some experts suggested that the graphic video would be unsuccessful in its aims to reduce drug taking by young people. Do you agree?

Alternative strategies include raising awareness and changing attitudes. In presenting information to people in order to promote change, Taylor (1995) suggests that it should:

- Be colourful, vivid, virtually statistics-free and use case histories
- Come from an expert source
- Discuss both sides of the issue
- Have the strongest arguments at the beginning and end of the message
- Be short and clear
- Have explicit rather than implicit conclusions
- Not be too extreme.

> ### Reflective activity
>
> Consider promotional material you have distributed to patients or have seen in hospitals or your local doctor's surgery. To what extent does it fulfil the criteria suggested by Taylor (1995)?

Raising awareness

As we have seen in relation to many areas, such as hygiene (page 49) and nutrition (pages 51–58), the first step in encouraging improved health behaviour is to increase awareness of healthy and unhealthy options.

> ### Over to you
>
> Major campaigns have been launched to raise awareness of specific risks, such as AIDS and meningitis. Investigate such resources and consider the following questions. What kinds of messages are used to inform people? Do they impart knowledge? If so, does it relate to seriousness, vulnerability or other aspects of the disease? Does the information attempt to alter beliefs or attitudes? Do they try to influence subjective norms or people's perceptions, or their own behavioural control?

The two models of health behaviour we have considered, the health belief model (pages 58–64) and the theory of planned behaviour (pages 64–68), both suggest that awareness is important in promoting health behaviours. The HBM suggests that awareness is essential to making assessments of vulnerability and seriousness that combine to enable the individual to make judge of the threat posed by a disease. In addition, knowledge about the benefits of a particular health behaviour and ways to overcome barriers enable the individual to sway their cost–benefit analysis in favour of engaging in healthier behaviours.

Awareness is also important from the perspective of the TPB. Here, knowledge is a prerequisite in the formation of attitudes towards health behaviours. Inadequate awareness or misinformation would lead to poor health behaviour choices; therefore it is the role of health promotion to ensure that people are aware of sufficient and appropriate resources so that they can make informed choices.

> ### ☞ Over to you
>
> Return to the following descriptions of studies reported earlier in this chapter:
>
> ● Bernstein Hyman *et al.* 1994 (page 64)
> ● Hochbaum 1958 (page 58)
> ● Haefner and Kirscht 1970 (page 61)
> ● O'Brien and Lee 1990 (page 60)
> ● Rimer *et al.* 1991 (page 60).
>
> For each study, identify the nature of the information that the participants needed in order to improve their awareness of health risks and justify your explanation using either the HBM or the TPB.

Persuasive communication and changing attitudes

It is clear that awareness or understanding of issues alone is insufficient to guarantee an improvement in health behaviours. As both the HBM and the TPB show, changing behaviours is not a simple matter of increasing knowledge – effective health promotion must change beliefs or attitudes before behaviour change will occur. For example, Kirscht *et al.* (1978) found that threat messages about weight control in obese children (which should have induced a change in maternal attitude) did indeed affect behaviour (the children lost weight). This shows that attitudes can affect behaviour. However, Leventhal and Cleary (1980) failed to change health behaviour; even when smokers' attitudes were manipulated by stimulating feelings of vulnerability they did not stop smoking. Similarly, despite their coverage, television campaigns to reduce alcohol and drug abuse have been unsuccessful (Morrison *et al.* 1976). Hovland (based at Yale University) developed a theory of persuasive communication in the 1950s (the 'Yale model') that laid the foundation for modern theories of attitude change.

In order for a communication to be persuasive it must first be noticed, thus attention is the first stage of the model. Individuals are unlikely be influenced by 'Stop smoking' posters unless they are prominent. However, attending to the message alone does not guarantee attitude change, the recipient must also be able to understand the message. Comprehension is required for the persuasive attempt to be successful. For example, if a hospital wants its staff to adhere to a complex policy of segregating waste but this is not clearly explained, they are unlikely to follow the required procedure.

Whilst both attention and comprehension are necessary, they are not sufficient. Finally the message must be accepted. Acceptance does not necessarily demand belief but it does require that the receiver acts on their understanding. Thus, if we see a notice that says 'closing doors saves lives', we may not believe that the consequences of our actions will be that significant but, because we understand the sentiment of the message we have seen, our behaviours change accordingly.

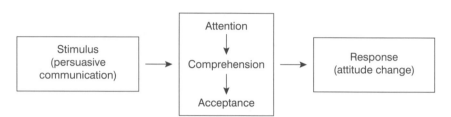

The Yale model of persuasive communication

This notion of a staged sequence in the processing of persuasive information is now referred to as systematic processing (McGuire 1969); it requires the receiver to engage in thinking about the message rather than being a passive recipient. To account for some of the observed effects of persuasive communication, the model has been adapted to incorporate more stages. McGuire (1968) separated 'acceptance' into two stages, yielding and retention, and introduced a final stage, action. This version differentiates between being persuaded by the message (yielding) and retaining that changed belief (retention). Patients with hypertension may see posters that advise them to cut down on salt and, although they understand and accept the message, they may forget after a while why it was important. Thus, initially behaviour changes, i.e. there is action, but this may revert to inaction when retention fails.

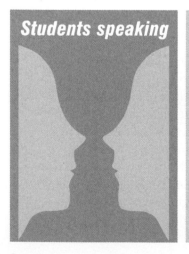

Students speaking

Patients who apparently understand the severity and seriousness of their condition and have cues to action may not always change their behaviour

A student nurse with experience of chronic care

Although I have cared for patients when they have needed amputation of toes, feet and limbs that relate to poor circulation, these patients often seem to view this as due to a mix of factors, rather just around their smoking. Once they have had their operation they are often very concerned about their other foot and take more care with this. However, they do not always give up smoking, and if they are diabetic they may not control their blood sugar any better even though they have already had one amputation.

Factors affecting persuasion

In addition to describing the process of behaviour change, the Yale model also indicates the factors that can influence the acceptance of attempted persuasive communication (Janis and Hovland 1959). These factors are:

- The communicator of the message – the role, affiliations and intentions of the source
- The content of the message – the topics, appeals, arguments and stylistic features
- The media characteristics of the message – whether interaction is direct or indirect and the sensory modality used
- The situational surroundings – such as the social setting and extraneous pleasant or unpleasant stimuli
- The characteristics of the recipient – such as persuadability and self-confidence (Janis and Field 1959).

Communicator factors

The source of the message is an important factor in the success of attitude change. Some key factors include:

- The credibility and expertise of the source – communicators who are believable and perceived to be knowledgeable in their field are more effective
- Communicators who argue against their own best interests – a nutritionist who says it is OK to eat some saturated fat is more likely to be believed than a dairy farmer who says the same thing
- Attractiveness of the communicator – Chaiken (1979) asked students to persuade others to sign a petition; physically attractive individuals were more effective
- Perceived similarity of the communicator to the recipient – this is particularly so if the similarity is deemed to be relevant to the issue
- Likeability of the source – we are more readily persuaded by an individual whom we find pleasant than one we do not.

Content factors

Many characteristics of the message are also important, these include:

- **Emotional content** – is it fear-arousing?
- **Medium** – verbal or visual?
- **Argument** – is it presented as a one-sided or two-sided debate?

Fear-arousing arguments may be effective, although a range of factors affect the likelihood of recipients adhering to the message. Rogers (1975) suggested that these were: the unpleasantness of the fear-arousing suggestion; the probability of the event occurring if the recommendation is not followed; and the perceived effectiveness of the recommended action. Persuasive communication should therefore be most powerful if the recipient finds the suggestion relatively unpleasant, really believes it will happen and expects that the evasive action will be effective.

However, it is not always the case that high levels of fear-arousal are the most effective. Janis and Feshbach (1953) (page 50) found the reverse, with low levels of fear-arousal producing the most behaviour change. Thus, health messages about, for example, skin cancer and sun bathing that focus on avoiding wrinkles and getting sunburn may be more effective than threats about dying of cancer.

Some additional factors have been shown to affect attitude change. Howard (1997) found that familiarity had a powerful influence. Students were more likely to be persuaded by an argument couched in familiar terms, such as 'Don't put all your eggs in one basket' or 'Don't bury your head in the sand', than one expressed in phrases such as 'Don't pretend a problem doesn't exist'.

Media factors

For messages geared towards encouraging healthy behaviour, which medium is most effective – or does the efficacy of the communication depend on the message being conveyed?

The answer seems to depend on the stage at which the recipient is likely to resist the message. If difficulties are likely to arise at the comprehension stage, for instance if the message is complex, then written communications appear to be most effective. However, where problems arise with yielding to the message, more direct media, such as face-to-face interactions, are more effective (Chaiken and Eagly 1976).

Thus, explaining the impact of high- and low-density lipoproteins on cholesterol levels would be better presented on paper, since it is a relatively complex issue. In contrast, persuading school children to eat five portions of fruit or vegetables a day would be more successfully tackled face to face, as the problem is not one of difficulty with comprehension but of encouraging participation.

Situational factors

Presenting a communication as either a one- or two-sided argument can be advantageous in different situations. Where views are likely to be unopposed, a one-sided argument will achieve opinion change more quickly, if only temporarily. However, in many health-related situations, one view is likely to be countered by another: non-smokers by smokers for example. In these instances, persuasive communication is more likely to be effective if both sides of the argument are acknowledged.

In these instances, primacy and recency effects come into play (see page 101). If the time lag between the presentation of the two sides of the issue is small, the first message should be more effective (because of the primacy effect). If, however, the interval is long, the later message will be better remembered, because of the recency effect, so is likely to result in greater attitude change (Petty and Cacioppo 1981).

So, in a heated debate in a trust meeting about the merits of foundation status, the first speaker is advantaged because the presentations are likely to follow one another in quick succession. However, if cases are to be presented in a monthly bulletin in successive editions, there is a distinct advantage in being the last to appear.

Reflective activity

A local community group is campaigning for the loan of medical equipment such as wheelchairs and transcutaneous electrical neurological stimulation (TENS) machines to be free but this is being opposed by health centre managers. If you represented either the local community group or the health centre management and could design screen savers to appear on every local library computer monitor for one week, would your message be more persuasive if it appeared for the first week or the second? If each group were allocated an afternoon to give presentations to the residents' association, would you rather speak first or last? If your message were complex, would you opt for the verbal presentation or a written message on the computers?

Another situational factor affecting the persuasiveness of communication is the nature of the distractions with which it has to compete. It seems obvious that a message will be less effective if it is in competition with other stimuli for the recipient's attention, but this is not always the case. This is because distractions prevent rehearsal and therefore impair memory. While a viewpoint with which an individual agrees may be disadvantaged by interruptions (they are less able to focus on the additional supporting arguments), a contrary viewpoint may benefit from distractions. If an individual is attending to a message that conflicts with their prevailing view, but is distracted, they will be unable to generate their own arguments against it; thus it will seem more persuasive.

AIDS education programmes

Acquired immune deficiency syndrome (AIDS) is a condition diagnosed by the presence of specific secondary diseases caused by infection with HIV, which destroys helper T cells, part of the body's defence system (see page 132). Infection with HIV makes the body vulnerable to the secondary diseases that characterise AIDS, such as pneumonia caused by *Pneumocystis carinii* and the rare skin cancer Kaposi's sarcoma, in addition to causing a complex of symptoms, including fever and fatigue.

There may be a long period of incubation of HIV, commonly 5–8 years, without the appearance of any symptoms associated with the infection. During this time, and subsequently, the infected individual presents a health risk to others if (and only if) they engage in behaviours that can transmit the virus. These include activities in which infected bodily fluids (blood or semen) can pass between individuals. Vaginal, anal and oral sex all carry such risks, as does the sharing of needles and syringes for injection of drugs. Physical contact, kissing, sharing crockery and contact with tears and saliva do not represent a threat to health.

Since infectious individuals may be unaware of their status, all people exposed to routes of infection are at risk and should engage in health-protective behaviours.

Treatments for AIDS are being developed but prevention continues to be the best strategy for promoting health in this context. However, most evidence suggests that the health promotion programmes attempted so far have been largely unsuccessful. Worldwide the number of infected individuals is still increasing and, although infection in the UK appears to have reached a plateau, more people are still becoming infected.

One group for whom the risk of infection is still increasing is intravenous drug users, because blood contact via non-sterile equipment is a route to infection (see page 50). They are therefore a key target for health education programmes. The development of such programmes has much to learn from the failure of early campaigns.

When awareness of AIDS first emerged in the early 1980s the highest risk groups were considered to be homosexual males and intravenous drug users. Unprotected sexual intercourse carries a high risk of transmission (especially for the recipient) so early campaigns used fear-arousing appeals to attempt to encourage safer practices, emphasising non-penetrative sex and reducing the number of sexual partners. The campaigns relied on posters, leaflet drops to households and information provided via television, radio and print media.

Despite the high profile of these campaigns, young people still reported a sense of invulnerability to HIV. The campaigns did result in some increase in knowledge about HIV and AIDS but this was not always accurate, as lay beliefs and stereotypes affected the way in which people interpreted new information. So, although considerable information was available, few people altered their behaviour. Woodcock *et al.* (1992) reported that participants offered justifications for high-risk behaviours such as believing that the risk of AIDS had been blown out of proportion or that their partners were not promiscuous.

Temoshok *et al.* (1987) compared gay, bisexual and heterosexual men's beliefs about HIV. The gay and bisexual men had higher levels of knowledge about HIV than heterosexual men and some studies have found a change in the behaviour of gay and bisexual men to reduce risk (e.g. Curran *et al.* 1985), although many continued with unsafe sex (Kelly *et al.* 1990). In contrast, no change was identified by Simkins and Ebenhage (1984) in the heterosexual population.

More recent campaigns have concentrated on safer sex and the use of condoms as a barrier against HIV infection. Importantly, they have also attempted to change the behaviour of heterosexuals, who are currently the fastest growing risk group. The World Health Organization estimates that more than 90% of new HIV infections are the result of heterosexual transmission.

The General Household Survey, comparing British households between 1983 and 1991, indicated a small increase in the use of condoms, especially by younger people.

One reason for the reluctance of heterosexuals to change their behaviour is the mistaken belief that AIDS is limited to minority groups (homosexuals or intravenous drug users). This myth of invulnerability results in people denying that they are at risk and so failing to alter their health behaviours appropriately. Another consequence of the myth is that it perpetuates a climate of blame directed at those groups and a stigmatisation of people with AIDS (Pitts and Phillips 1998).

👉 *Over to you*

The governmental consultation paper *Our Healthier Nation* states, under the heading 'publicity campaigns' that: 'The Government will continue to use publicity campaigns on issues such as occupational health, road safety, drink-driving, anti-drugs initiatives, safe sex and smoking' (pages 34–35).

Design a publicity campaign on one of the topics listed above using the ideas in this chapter. Write an accompanying document to the government justifying your choice of strategies.

Social skills training

Social skills training can be used as a primary prevention measure to enable people to identify their personal and social needs and to develop the skills required to meet those health needs. For instance, many smokers report that they smoke in order to reduce social anxiety, so finding alternative means to relax could be beneficial. Since the largest group of new smokers is young people, they need to be equipped with the necessary social skills to avoid taking up smoking at all. This can be achieved by teaching relaxation techniques, so allowing individuals alternatives to smoking for coping with difficult social situations. Self-management strategies used with smokers encourage the participant to monitor the circumstances under which smoking occurs. Self-reward techniques can then be used to separate smoking behaviour from the environmental cues with which it is associated.

Social skills training can be used not only to cope with emotional consequences of the social environment but also to impart practical social skills. Bachman *et al.* (1988) used social skills training to teach young people to say 'no' to drugs. Students were encouraged to talk to each other about drugs, to state their disapproval of drug taking and to say that they did not take drugs. The aim was to create a new anti-drug-taking social norm and to give the participants experience of refusing drugs. The programme succeeded in changing attitudes to drugs and reducing cannabis use.

> ## Over to you
>
> Abraham and Sheeran (1993) recommended the use of skills training to encourage safer sex. They suggested teaching skills that young people could use in the following contexts:
>
> - Buying condoms
> - Negotiating condom use with a partner
> - Use of condoms.
>
> Furthermore, several teaching strategies were proposed, including:
>
> - Tuition
> - Role-play
> - Feedback
> - Modelling
> - Practice.
>
> Using the ideas of contexts and teaching strategies suggested by Abraham and Sheeran (1993), devise ways to teach young people about either healthy nutrition or an aspect of hygiene.

Kelly *et al.* (1989) employed a behavioural intervention with a group of gay men. This included risk reduction information as well as social skills training in sexual assertiveness and the promotion of social support groups to discourage high-risk behaviours. Compared to controls on a waiting list, those who were randomly assigned to participate reported greatly reduced unsafe sexual behaviours and this change had been maintained by the follow-up 8 months later.

Self-empowerment

Self-empowerment models of health promotion offer an alternative strategy to that proposed by social cognition theories (such as the HBM and TPB). The aim of the self-empowerment approach is to give the individual the information and skills to make healthy choices through an ability to control their physical, social and internal environments (Marks *et al.* 2000). In addition to skills training other techniques employed include assertiveness training, group work, problem solving and educational drama. This technique has been used with young people in a range of HIV-preventative interventions. The techniques used by Abraham and Sheeran (1994) included:

- Rehearsing the interactions involved in situations such as buying condoms
- Rehearsing the possible interactions in sexual negotiations
- Questioning sexual scripts where negotiation is prevented
- Peer education programmes
- Programmes aimed to identify and overcome personal obstacles to HIV prevention.

Such initiatives, Abraham and Sheeran argue, offer the opportunity to develop skills and promote self-efficacy, which is a good predictor of behavioural intention and behaviour (Bandura 1992). This technique probably offers a more powerful approach than simply providing information to raise awareness or attempting to manipulate attitudes.

> ### Over to you
>
> Find out about World AIDS Day or AIDS Awareness Week health campaigns, using the Internet or local health promotion resources. Consider the way the materials used have been designed; use the Health Belief Model or Theory of Planned Behaviour to justify their approaches. Plan a programme for raising AIDS awareness and prepare a briefing document explaining the strategies you would like to employ.

One disadvantage of successful public campaigns is that, by making people aware of their responsibility for their own health, health education may be engendering a culture of blame (Stroebe 2000). Information fuels arguments such as 'I've looked after myself and am healthy; you are ill, therefore it must be your own fault'. This is characteristic of the effects of AIDS campaigns.

Smoking education programmes

A range of strategies have been used in an attempt to help young people to avoid taking up smoking and to help those people who wish to quit. These focus on trying to change behaviour. Many smokers report that they smoke in order to reduce social anxiety, so finding alternative means to relax could be beneficial. Since the largest group of new smokers is young people, they need to be equipped with the necessary social skills to avoid taking up smoking at all. This can be achieved by teaching relaxation techniques, so allowing individuals alternatives to smoking for coping with difficult social situations.

Self-management strategies used with smokers encourage the participant to monitor the circumstances under which smoking occurs. Self-reward techniques can then be used to separate smoking behaviour from the environmental cues with which it is associated. Although behaviour change may be achieved by these techniques, unless this is accompanied by a change in beliefs, the new behaviour may not be sustained.

Anti-smoking campaigns

Anti-smoking campaigns aim to change attitudes and may do so but do not necessarily succeed in changing behaviour as a consequence. They encourage people to want to give up but do not increase success. They do, however, have some benefits. They provide information – most smokers now know smoking is bad for them – and have instilled an anti-smoking attitude in the general population that can help smokers who are trying to quit. When many smokers, affected by the same advertising campaign, decide to quit together they create for themselves a supportive social network, which is central to their success. Advertising campaigns are also important in stopping non-smoking adults from taking up the habit (Warner and Murt 1982).

Prevention programmes

Whilst advertising campaigns may be effective in stopping the potential adult smoker, these individuals have already managed to resist smoking during adolescence. Why do increasing numbers of young people still take up smoking despite their early exposure to dissuasive material?

Effectiveness of prevention programmes may depend on their timing. The concept of a window of vulnerability suggests that there is an age at which children or young adults are likely to begin to abuse drugs. For nicotine dependence, this occurs when children are first exposed to their peers smoking. School anti-smoking campaigns should therefore target this age group.

Workplace smoking

Prevention can also be exercised through banning smoking. Smoking bans are typical of hospitals, surgeries and educational buildings. Parry *et al.* (2000) investigated the effectiveness of a smoking ban implemented in a Scottish university. The potential benefits of such a ban would be to:

- Reduce opportunities for smokers to smoke so they might cut down
- Protect non-smokers from the effects of passive smoking
- Reduce smoking-related litter.

Bans may either restrict areas available for smoking, for instance by providing a designated area, or prohibit smoking within the buildings. The latter was chosen in this case.

The result, however, was that smokers congregated at entrances (where littering increased) and, as a result, the profile of smoking within the university was raised rather than lowered. In addition, perceived discrimination against smokers resulted in increased sympathy for them. So, while the objective of improving air quality inside the buildings had been achieved, any reduction in smoking by staff needed to be approached in a different way.

Social inoculation

Evans *et al.* (1988) proposed social influence intervention as a preventative measure to reduce uptake of smoking by school children. This suggests that smoking is acquired, at least in part, by modelling the behaviour of others. When children see other individuals apparently enjoying what they know to be high-risk behaviours, their fears are reduced and the potential positive consequences are enhanced. To counter this, children should be exposed to high-status, non-smoking models (Evans 1976). This would be more effective in a context of behavioural inoculation. This, like vaccination, exposes the individual to a weakened dose of the offending agent in order for them to develop resistance against it. In this context children could be allowed to develop their own (strong) counter-arguments against a (weak) message in favour of drug use.

Taking smoking as an example, three stages follow from Evans's social influence intervention programme.

- Information about the negative effects of smoking should be presented in a way that appeals to adolescents. This needs to focus on the immediate disadvantages, which are tangible to teenagers, such as smelling of smoke, being unpleasant to kiss, having yellow fingers or the cost (i.e. raise perception of barriers).

- Positive images of non-smokers must convey independence and self-reliance. These raise adolescents' expectations of themselves as independent thinkers while depicting smokers as vulnerable to advertising (i.e. raise perception of benefits).

- The peer group should facilitate non-smoking rather than smoking. This can be achieved using older, respected, non-smoking students to convey information about how to resist the temptation to smoke when invited (i.e. alter subjective norms).

In assessing the effectiveness of such programmes, Elder *et al.* (1993) found that the participants had learned how to refuse cigarettes but this did not relate to cigarette use – in other words the adolescents had learned how to say no but continued to smoke. Flay *et al.* (1992) suggest that intervention programmes are only effective in stopping experimental smokers, who would cease of their own accord anyway. They do not tackle the problem of those destined to become adult smokers.

An alternative is to teach life skills, enhancing the self-esteem of adolescents in order to bolster their ability to resist peer pressure to smoke. This technique appears to be as effective as intervention programmes (Botvin *et al.* 1980).

An application of Flay's inoculation model employed in the USA is peer resistance training. This aims to help children to resist pressure to use drugs by teaching refusal skills and reinforcing group norms against drug abuse. Benefits from such schemes include improved self-esteem and communication and delayed onset of alcohol, cigarette and cannabis use. However, these initial gains tend not to persist for longer than a year (McAlister *et al.* 1980). In Britain, peer education is used to encourage youngsters to take responsibility to achieve and sustain a drug-free lifestyle. Messages from peers are arguably more acceptable to young people than more traditional health education from adults (Quirk *et al.* 1993).

Key points   *Top tips*

- Mass media appeals can reach large numbers of people, although they are not always successful

- Campaigns may fail because people are unwilling to believe that they are vulnerable to health risks and even when people accept the existence of health risks this may not be sufficient to motivate a change in behaviour

- Research suggests that campaigns should identify a focus (such as reducing barriers or changing subjective norms) based on the target group rather than just providing information about dangers.

Conclusions

Primary prevention strategies aim to encourage positive health behaviours by providing information that warns of risks to health without inducing fear. Such strategies can be used to improve health behaviours relating to hygiene and nutrition. In the case of healthy eating, biological explanations suggest that genetic factors, such as the predisposition to obesity, affect our health. Metabolic rate, fat cells and weight all appear to have inherited components. Eating habits may also be acquired, by classical or operant conditioning and through social learning. Foods may become associated with emotional states and may act as a reinforcer (or punisher). We may imitate the amount or types of food that role models consume. Cultural factors may determine aspects of health behaviours such as the types of food we eat and when we eat them.

The health belief model attempts to explain health behaviours by considering the way in which we process information relating to health issues. It suggests that, in relation to any health behaviour, we have five central beliefs about our vulnerability, the seriousness of the condition, potential barriers to and benefits of taking evasive action and cues that trigger the behaviour. When these variables favour action over inaction, positive health behaviour should occur. This explanation can successfully account for preventative behaviours such as immunisations and self-examination and for attendance or non-attendance at screening tests.

The theory of planned behaviour suggests that health behaviours are determined by the intention to act and the extent of perceived behavioural control. When an individual both intends to engage in a health behaviour and feels that they have the power to do so, they will take action. Intention is determined by factors such as knowledge, attitudes and subjective norms while perceived behavioural control may be affected by self-efficacy as well as intrinsic motivation and external factors. The theory can help to direct health campaigns by identifying why people fail to engage in health behaviours, for example to promote breast feeding or condom use.

Health education programmes can therefore be based on the findings of research, not only on the success of previous campaigns but also on the predictions of the HBM and the TPB. In addition to, and perhaps more importantly than, providing information to raise awareness, health promotion programmes need to change attitudes to health and health behaviours.

> ## Over to you
>
> Consider how you would develop and test your own health education strategy, based on either the health belief model or the theory of planned behaviour. Once you have decided on a health behaviour to promote, it may help to draw out a large copy of the model (as on page 65), inserting the factors that you think are relevant to the issue you are exploring.

RRRRRRapid recap

Check your progress so far by working through each of the following questions.

1. What are the key elements in the theory of planned behaviour?
2. The following factors could affect an individual who is thinking about giving up smoking: the existence of many non-smoking restaurants; the belief that smoky clothes is unpleasant; a desire to combat the effects of smoking on their asthma; the knowledge that they can stop themselves from starting again once they have said they've given up. Explain which of these factors would relate to each aspect of the theory of planned behaviour.

If you have difficulty with either of the questions, read through the section again to refresh your understanding before moving on.

Key references

Other references are in the main reference list at the end of the book.

Abraham, C., Sheeran, P., Spears, R. and Abrams, D. (1992) Health beliefs and the promotion of HIV-preventative infections among teenagers: a Scottish perspective. *Health Psychology*, **11**: 363–370.

Murray, M. and McMillan, C. (1993) Health beliefs, locus of control, emotional control and women's cancer screening behaviour. *British Journal of Clinical Psychology*, **32**: 87–100.

Pitts, M. and Phillips, K. (1998) *The Psychology of Health: An introduction*. Routledge, London.

Reddy, C.V. (1989) Parents' beliefs about vaccination. *British Medical Journal*, **299**: 739.

Rutter, D.R. (2000) Attendance and reattendance for breast cancer screening: a prospective 3-year test of the theory of planned behaviour. *British Journal of Health Psychology*, **5**: 1–13.

Walker, J. (2001) *Control and the Psychology of Health*. Open University Press, Buckingham.

3

Adherence to treatment

Learning outcomes

By the end of this chapter you should be able to:

- Explain what is meant by patient non-adherence

- Describe and evaluate methods for assessing adherence

- Explain patient-related factors that help to understand why patients may not follow instructions given to them by health professionals

- Explain practitioner-related factors that help to understand why patients may not follow instructions given to them by health professionals

- Identify and justify good practice that would help patients to understand, remember and act on advice.

Patients receiving treatment from their health care providers are exposed to information. This can vary from relatively simple details about when and how to take medicine prescribed by the GP to complex anatomical information relating to a serious illness and possible treatment options. The patients must comprehend and remember this information and then act on it. The advice they are given for action may include not just drug regimes but instructions on diet, abstaining from or reducing smoking or alcohol consumption, taking rest or exercise, avoiding stress and attending future appointments. In many cases, patients do not follow these instructions. In this chapter we explore the reasons why patients may fail to follow medical advice and look at how this problem may be reduced.

Is non-adherence a problem?

Early research in this area referred to *compliance* with medical advice, implying that non-compliant patients were being deliberately 'disobedient' when they failed to follow instructions. This is now being replaced with the term *adherence*, suggesting that the patient may, or may not, 'stick to' the advice given. This is preferable as it recognises that:

- Patients have choices and may be opting not to follow instructions

- When patients do not follow advice, the reason may be because they cannot rather than they will not

- Patient–practitioner communication is a co-operative process rather than a one-way channel.

Even when patients believe that they are adhering to treatment, this may not be the case . . .

Out-patient pre-operative clinics – a student's observations

A lady came into the pre-assessment clinic. During her previous admission a few months ago she had been instructed to eat a low-fat diet, prior to having removal of her gall bladder (cholecystectomy). She had been handling pain during this time, and said she had been sticking to a low fat diet, but when the pre-admission nurse at the clinic questioned what she had been eating she had not understood what this type of diet should really be. Despite this, she had lost weight.

Many patients do not adhere to the advice they are given, although estimates of non-adherence rates vary with patient group, research method and definition of adherence. Ley and Llewelyn (1995) provide a comparison of reported non-adherence rates in different medical settings and for a range of types of advice obtained from different research sources. The results demonstrate a considerable problem, with non-adherence being consistently high, ranging from 39.5% to 60%. Such findings suggest that patients are not benefiting as much as they could from the information and follow-up care provided for them by health professionals.

This behaviour has the potential to cause pain, distress and fatalities in patients. For example, Abram *et al.* (1971) estimated that in 4% of haemodialysis patients with end-stage renal disease, failure to adhere to dietary advice was the direct cause of death. In addition, non-adherence has indirect costs in terms of wasted drugs and the need for re-admission to hospital. Ausburn (1981) estimated that 20–25% of cases of hospitalisation were likely to be due to failure to follow the appropriate regime for taking medication.

Non-adherence by health professionals

This chapter focuses on the investigation of non-adherence of patients to the advice of their health care workers but do they themselves practise what they preach? Apparently not! Forsythe *et al.* (1999) surveyed over 1000 British consultants and GPs and asked them about their adherence to good practice guidelines. It is recommended that doctors do not prescribe medication for themselves or their immediate families but over 70% reported that they failed to adhere to this advice and would self-prescribe.

Similarly, over 80% reported treating and prescribing medication for members of their own family even though this is in contravention of the British Medical Association guidelines.

Neither, it seems, do health care professionals always follow recommended protocol in the treatment of other patients. In a study of the care of breast cancer patients, Schleifer *et al.* (1991) found that 56% experienced changes to their chemotherapy medications that were unjustified. Similarly, Yoong *et al.* (1992) showed that, in their examinations of pregnant women, obstetricians were failing to follow more than three-quarters of departmental protocols.

Health care professionals have a commitment to maintain their professional education; failure to do so is another example of non-compliance. Nevertheless, O'Brien (1997) reported that approximately 40% of doctors are underinformed because they do not fulfil their ongoing training requirements and those who do not update their training are less likely to request appropriate screening tests for their patients.

Non-adherence also affects health care professionals' own safety. O'Brien (1997) found that approximately 50% of medical students and hospital staff did not comply with procedures designed to protect them from infection when working with patients who were HIV-positive even though they perceived themselves to be at risk. She also found that, in one hospital, only 2% of doctors and nurses followed the recommendation to have an influenza vaccination.

Finally, O'Brien (1997) observes that, as with patients, improving compliance in health care professionals is difficult. Providing information is not sufficient to improve adherence, although memory aids and behavioural strategies are effective.

When non-adherence is good for you

When non-adherence arises because the patient judges that adherence is not in their best interests, they have made a rational judgement; hence this is referred to as rational non-adherence. Patients making the decision not to follow advice may not, in some instances, be putting themselves at significant risk. For example, effort spent on absolute adherence to diabetic control measures may only reduce the risk of serious complications rather than guaranteeing recovery or even relief from symptoms (Cahill *et al.* 1976).

Patients may judge the possible benefits of compliance – such as the risk of dependence, side effects, time and effort – against the expected benefits – such as symptom relief. Donovan and Blake

(1992) observed that patients may therefore opt not to comply as a result of their reasoning.

Measuring adherence

There are many different ways of studying whether patients are following advice, the commonest being to ask the patients themselves. Others include practitioner reports, observation by other people (such as family), physical records (such as pill counts) and physiological measures (such as blood tests for the presence of medicines). Each of these is discussed below.

Asking patients and health professionals

The simplest and most frequently used technique for studying adherence is the patient-report. When asked to gauge how closely they have followed the advice they were given, their responses are not, however, entirely reliable. Patients tend to misreport their compliance, underestimating non-compliance and overestimating compliant behaviours. This may be either because they are hiding the truth in order to avoid disapproval or because they are simply unaware of their own behaviour. As we will see, both understanding of and memory for medical information may be faulty; if so, it is unlikely that a patient's own judgement of their adherence is a reliable source of evidence. Roth (1987) compared the findings of several studies and concluded that patient self-reporting of adherence could not be corroborated by evidence from other measures.

Since self-reporting is the most common measure, it is important that efforts are made to maximise the reliability of data obtained by this method. Kaplan and Simon (1990) suggest that, if the questions asked are direct and simple, self-reporting can be used successfully.

Practitioner reporting can also be used but health care professionals, like patients, are inaccurate – possibly even more so, according to Ley (1988) – and Blackwell (1997) suggested that the estimates of compliance made by doctors and other health care professionals was little better than chance. For example, Finney *et al.* (1993) compared predictions made by primary health carers about the adherence of parents to children's short-term antibiotic treatment against objective measures of adherence (the amount of medication used and attendance at a follow-up appointment). The health carer's predictions considerably overestimated parental adherence.

media watch

Poor recall mars research and treatment

'How many of you didn't floss your teeth this morning?' said psychologist Cynthia Rand, PhD, to an auditorium full of researchers and clinicians.

Few were willing to admit they hadn't. Yet they were a group that relies on accurate self-reports for their livelihoods.

With her question, Rand highlighted one of the many problems with self-report data: people don't like to admit they engage in socially undesirable behaviours. They also may lie about sensitive issues such as sex, drug use or abortions. And, far too often, people simply don't remember correctly because they never stored the information to begin with, their stored memory has become distorted or they can't retrieve the relevant information.

False reports can be costly and dangerous. For social and behavioural research, false reports can lead to faulty conclusions. For clinicians, they can lead to inaccurate diagnoses. And for treatment adherence studies they can mean that the true cause of treatment failure may not be identified; successful treatment may be judged ineffective; costly diagnostic procedures may be ordered to re-evaluate the problem; and dose-response relationships may be miscalculated.

Fallible memories

One of the most significant problems with self-report stems from the fallible nature of human memory. Memory for specific events declines with time and the ability to retrieve memories often depends on how they were encoded in the first place.

For example, people tend to retain details of unique stimulating and emotional events, said psychologist Roger Tourangeau. Unfortunately, researchers and clinicians are often interested in events the average person pays little attention to. Even something as seemingly important as taking a child for immunisations gets muddled in parents' minds: Tourangeau and his colleagues tested parents' ability to remember which immunisations their children had received as they left an immunisation clinic with their children. They then compared parent reports to clinic records.

Parents didn't do much better than chance. 'They had very poor memory for what happened,' said Tourangeau. That's because the event wasn't very memorable – it happened quickly and doctors use technical terms that are hard to remember. For this reason, researchers shouldn't use self-report for those unexciting events people are not likely to encode into memory, he said.

One way to get around memory problems is having participants keep daily diaries. But diaries are not foolproof either because participants often forget to fill them out and may even fake entries, said psychologist Saul Shiffman.

To combat these problems in studies of smoking, eating and stress, he uses small, palm-top computers that record the date and time when participants enter data and beep participants to remind them to input data. In smoking studies, participants carry the computers around with them and record each time they smoke. Five times a day, after a person records smoking a cigarette, the computer asks a series of questions about where they smoked and their mood while they smoked.

When Shiffman compared the moment-to-moment computer data with information participants provided on a retrospective questionnaire for the same time frame, he found no correlation. People were terrible at remembering where they smoked and their mood while they smoked.

continued

Shiffman highlighted another potential problem with self-report when he used the computers to examine smoking relapse in people who successfully completed a smoking-cessation programme. His work found that participants tended to report stereotypical ideas rather than true memories. In the experiments, the computers beeped participants several times a day and asked about their location, mood and whether they'd had a cigarette. Seventy days after they relapsed, Shiffman and his colleagues asked participants who had relapsed to describe their relapse experience. Their reports were inconsistent with their daily computer records. Instead, their descriptions matched those of non-smokers who were asked to guess what might trigger a smoking relapse.

Judgement calls?

People may also shy away from telling the truth if questions involve personally sensitive or potentially embarrassing issues such as abortion, drug use and sexual behaviour. Turner found that interviews conducted by computer can increase people's willingness to answer sensitive questions.

For example, adolescent boys were four times more likely to report same-sex intercourse to a computerised interviewer than on a paper-and-pencil questionnaire, Turner and his colleagues found. However, even with this dramatic increase, their reports did not approach the levels of adolescent same-sex contact retrospectively reported by adult men, said Turner.

But these techniques may not solve another problem with self-report: participants' desires to please the interviewer. Rand [is] particularly interested in [the] self-report of treatment adherence: she's found that people often tell clinicians they're following a treatment regimen when they're not.

Rand and her colleagues have electronically monitored how often people with asthma use their inhalers, using a computer chip that records each time the inhaler is activated. When people know doctors are monitoring their drug use, they self-report accurately. When they don't know, they tend to over-report treatment adherence.

But checking adherence isn't always enough. If patients know physicians will count their pills or weigh their inhaler canisters, they may 'dump' large portions of unused medicine. In Rand's inhaler study, about 14% of participants who didn't know they were being electronically monitored dumped medication from their inhalers – activating them up to 100 times an hour the day before their follow-up visit.

By Beth Azar (edited from *The APA Monitor*, 28(1), January 1997)

Asking others

Other individuals, such as family members, can be asked to monitor adherence, which has the advantage that they may be more objective and less intrusive. However, there are two problems with this technique. First, the observer is unlikely to be able to achieve non-stop monitoring so, for non-compliance such as smoking, drinking alcohol or eating disallowed foods, the assessment may be invalid. Secondly, the mere knowledge that behaviours are being observed may affect the patient's compliance, creating an artificial situation (in which the patient is probably more likely to comply). While this may be desirable in terms of their health, the observation is less accurate.

Physical and physiological measures

Mechanical techniques, such as pill pots that record the number of times they have been opened (e.g. Cramer *et al.* 1989) and relaxation tapes that identify when they have been played, provide a way to verify the accuracy of other methods. However, just because a pill pot has been opened or a taped played does not guarantee that the medicine has been taken at the right time (if at all) or the tape listened to; therefore even more sophisticated techniques may provide less than accurate data.

Finally, physiological measures of patients, e.g. biochemical indicators of medicine use in the blood or urine, can be taken. These measures of compliant behaviour are expensive, inconsistent between individuals and can only detect whether a drug has been taken, not whether it was taken at the right time or in the correct quantity. Their use is also limited to those individuals who are sufficiently compliant to turn up to be tested. However, Roth (1987) suggests that these measures are more reliable than counting pills, so they may be of use. For example, Wysocki *et al.* (1989) found that use of a glucometer for self-monitoring of blood glucose by diabetics produced a short-term increase in compliance but that this effect was rapidly lost unless it was combined with another source of motivation, in this case a behavioural contract.

Key points   Top tips

- Non-adherence by patients is common, with perhaps more than 50% of patients not following advice given
- Non-adherence may be rational and deliberate, or unintentional
- Health professionals also demonstrate non-adherence in relation to work guidelines and regulations
- Adherence may be measured in a variety of different ways, each of which has possible problems and potential inaccuracies.

Predicting and explaining adherence and non-adherence

There are several possible reasons why patients may not follow medical advice that they have been given. These include:

- Not being aware of the information (e.g. if they have not listened advice or looked at a leaflet)
- Being unable to understand the advice, so unable to follow it

- Not believing advice to be true, or to be relevant to themselves
- Not being able to recall the information in order to follow it
- Not having the motivation to persist with following advice
- Being unable to cope with the requirements of following the advice
- Choosing to ignore advice or to follow a different course of action.

There are several theories that can help us to understand the causes of adherence and how it may be increased. In this chapter we will consider a behavioural and a cognitive model of compliance, two models of memory, the parallel response model and also the two models of health behaviour discussed in Chapter 2. Each of these helps us to understand a different aspect of adherence.

The behavioural model of compliance

One explanation for the acquisition and performance – or otherwise – of behaviours is operant conditioning. This theory of learning forms the basis for the behavioural model of compliance. The major proponent of operant conditioning, B.F. Skinner, identified several key mechanisms that determine whether behaviours are repeated. He suggested that an individual (human or animal) performs a random variety of behaviours and, of those, some are reinforced (result in pleasant consequences that increase the frequency of the behaviour) while others are punished (result in unpleasant consequences that decrease the frequency of the behaviour). These behaviours may be responses to certain stimuli or cues in the environment.

Reinforcement in the context of adherence to medical advice most obviously includes health benefits such as reduction in pain or other unpleasant symptoms (this type of reinforcement, in which good consequences derive from the removal of something unpleasant, is called negative reinforcement). An example of negative reinforcement can be seen in the relief a patient feels when their health improves and they no longer feel a burden to others – the removal of that pressure feels good so acts as a reinforcer to promote further improvement. Other reinforcers could include praise from a health practitioner, feeling more energetic or losing weight. As these are good experiences, they are examples of positive reinforcement.

A technique called shaping, also based on operant conditioning, can be used to modify behaviours. This employs positive reinforcement to reward behaviours that more closely resemble the desired outcome. For example, patients with hypertension could be rewarded for progressively excluding unsuitable foods from their diet. Initially they would be reinforced for making straightforward adjustments to their diet such as changes to LoSalt, then subsequently for making more difficult refinements to their intake such as altering the way that they cook individual meals.

Punishment is less effective than reinforcement as a way to change behaviour, in part because it offers no alternative behaviour, it simply aims to suppress the performance of an action. Punishers could include the fear induced by threats such as telling children their teeth will rot if they don't brush them. The unpleasant effects of failure to adhere to advice, such as the threats to health caused by smoking, cannot act as effective punishers as they are not contingent – they do not immediately follow the performance of the behaviour.

The behavioural model would therefore predict that adherence would be best when there are appropriate and contingent reinforcers for performing the behaviours advised and, possibly, if non-adherent behaviour is punished. In reality, there may be many instances in which the reverse in true. Adherence itself may require commitments or lifestyle changes that are undesirable, such as extra time spent preparing a special diet, having to eat less palatable (but healthier) food, swallowing foul-tasting medicine or taking exercise. In addition, medication may have side effects. These consequences, if perceived to be unpleasant, act as punishers so would tend to reduce the likelihood of compliance. Conversely, the potentially reinforcing benefits of adherence are unlikely to be immediate, or even short term. Therefore the consequences – even for good compliers – cannot act as positive reinforcers because their effects are not contingent upon the behaviours required by adherence. Indeed, for a patient for whom the sick role (see Chapter 4) has become a way of life, recovery – and therefore adherence – may represent a very frightening and powerful punisher.

media watch

Sisters can do it for themselves

It's the blight of every woman's three-year calendar. The smear test, that dreaded half-hour where we sit with our legs open as someone prods us with a metal speculum like something out of a medieval torture chamber: no surprise then that almost one-fifth of women neglect to have smears – and a significant majority choose not to because of the uncomfortable nature of the examination itself.

All women between 25 and 64 are recommended to have a Pap smear test every three years, a gynaecological examination that tests for cell changes in the cervix that may go on to become cervical cancer. The examination itself is straightforward but unpleasant: a metal speculum is inserted into the vagina to hold open the vaginal walls, while the doctor or nurse inserts a spatula to obtain a sample of cells from the cervix.

'We all know that women hate to have smears and of the certain proportion that don't turn up for smears at all, a fair number don't turn up because they hate the examination itself,' says Dr Anne Szarewski, clinical consultant at Cancer Research UK. 'We thought that if you could do a test at home in your own bathroom, it would be much less stressful and hopefully appeal to the women at the moment who are to scared to go for tests.'

According to Szarewski, studies so far have exclusively focused on the effectiveness of DIY kits without taking into consideration the very real anxiety and discomfort that the present method with its invasive speculum can cause. This is the first study of self-sampling which not only compares the effectiveness of self-sampling to clinical HPV tests and the existing Pap smear, but looks at the psychological element too: how do women feel about each of these different methods?

Although the NHS Cervical Screening Programme's target that 80% of eligible women are screened is being reached overall, the uptake is not consistent throughout the population. Women in inner-city areas are not attending in high levels, as well as women from certain ethnic groups who feel that being examined by men is culturally unacceptable. Another problem with the current smear is the anxiety caused by the high incidence of 'false positives'. Women who are detected to have 'cell abnormalities' turn out not to have cervical cancer. Research has shown that women with positive smear results experience high levels of anxiety, fear about cancer, and concerns about physical attractiveness and sexual function.

With experiences like this, it is hardly surprising that more women are choosing to stay away and bin their smear invites.

'So far previous studies looked at women using the kit while in the presence of the nurse which we think defeats the whole object', says Szarewski. 'One of the good points of HPV testing is that unlike the smear, when it tests negative it really is negative. We have all heard about women who have had negative smear tests and gone on to develop cervical cancer.'

For fans of self-sampling, the benefits are clear: to coax women who might otherwise avoid screening. Says Professor Sasieni [of Queen Mary College, London]: 'At the end of the day, self-sampling can encourage women who are not currently having smears to be screened. This has got to be an improvement'.

By Rebecca Hardy

Abridged from *The Independent Review* 12 January 2004, pages 4–5.

Reflective activity

In what ways do positive reinforcement and punishment affect the likelihood of women adhering to requests to attend smear tests or conducting self-sampling at home?

The behavioural model has the advantage that the effects of reinforcers and punishers on behaviour can be seen and, as such, measured. Consequently, the effectiveness of behavioural interventions is relatively easy to identify. However, the behavioural model gives us no insight into the thought processes that underlie adherent or non-adherent behaviour.

The cognitive model of compliance

Ley (1981) and Ley and Llewelyn (1995) have proposed a model that considers the patient's thinking and attempts to predict whether patients will comply with medical advice. It suggests that compliance or non-compliance is determined by three factors:

- Understanding
- Memory
- Satisfaction.

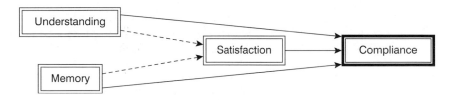

Ley's cognitive model of compliance

This is a cognitive model because it suggests that the determinants of compliance are processes related to *thinking*. According to the model, all three factors can affect compliance directly; better understanding and memory and greater satisfaction can each lead to a greater likelihood of compliance. In addition, the model suggests that patients who understand and remember the information that their health professional has supplied are more likely to be satisfied and, as an indirect consequence, are more likely to comply. These stages have been explored through research that we will consider in the following sections.

The role of understanding

We looked in detail at patient understanding in Chapter 2, so will consider it only briefly here. Parkin *et al.* (1976) reported that 49% of a sample of patients leaving hospital after treatment had little or no understanding of their illness and more than one-third were unclear about the drug regimen they were supposed to follow. Kerr *et al.* (2003) found that 39% of rectal cancer patients reported that there were aspects of communication with their clinician that were either incomprehensible or insufficient. This was particularly problematic for younger patients and those in larger hospitals. Armstrong *et al.* (1990) found little agreement between doctors and patients about whether or not a subsequent appointment had been recommended. Furthermore, Armstrong *et al.* reported that those patients who did not feel that the explanation they had been given was clear were less likely to adhere to recommendations. Evidence such as this suggests that a significant proportion of patients may not understand instructions and, as a consequence, cannot comply.

Patients who understand the information they are required to follow are more likely to adhere to it. For example, Ley *et al.* (1975) conducted an experiment to compare medication errors made by psychiatric patients using printed information that differed in difficulty. Those patients given leaflets with easier words and shorter sentences made fewer errors.

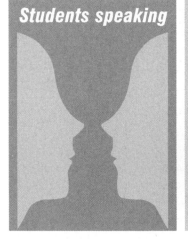

Students speaking

A key factor in empowering patients is ensuring that they understand their treatment . . .

An apprentice health care assistant

One old woman I was caring for had dementia, and was confused. She was due to have an operation to remove part of her colon, but it was really hard to get informed consent, because the doctor had to keep re-explaining the operation.

The relationship between understanding and compliance is not, however, always a simple one. Hamburg and Inoff (1982) studied adolescents with diabetes who were attending a summer camp and found an inverted U relationship – that is, adherence was worst for individuals with very poor or very good understanding of their condition and its treatment. It is possible that individuals with an intermediate level of knowledge are the best compliers because they have sufficient understanding to follow the advice but, because they are unaware of the long-term implications, they are less afraid so are not discouraged.

The role of satisfaction

Ley's model suggests that, although better understanding does result in improved compliance, this may be due in part to patient satisfaction. Patients whose doctors have enabled them to understand are more likely to be satisfied and satisfied patients are more likely to comply. DiMatteo *et al.* (1993) investigated compliance with medication, exercise and dietary advice given by doctors to patients with heart disease, diabetes and high blood pressure. Greater patient satisfaction correlated with better adherence to the advice and so, interestingly, did greater levels of job satisfaction in the doctors. It is worrying that the proportion of satisfied health care patients has remained fairly static over many years, despite efforts to improve levels of service (Ong *et al.* 1995). This lack of satisfaction will have a detrimental effect on motivation to comply.

The role of memory

 Keywords

Chronic
Persistent

One reason why patients may fail to adhere to medical advice is that they cannot remember it. For example, Kravitz *et al.* (1993) found that, although 90% of patients with a **chronic** condition could recall advice about medication, fewer remembered guidance about changes to their diet or exercise habits. Of those who did recall the advice, adherence ranged from 20% for adherence to recommendations about exercise to 90% for adherence to advice on medication.

In the following sections we will explore psychological explanations of memory and forgetting that can help us to understand why patients may forget what they are told. There have been many investigations studying patients' recall of medical information. These have used a range of techniques and sampled different groups of people. Such differences in approach have led to widely differing estimates of recall. Ley (1988) reviewed many such studies and found an overall average recall of around 50% with estimates from different sources ranging from 28% to 88%. Clearly a lot of patients forget a great deal of what has been communicated to them. Why is this?

Some factors seem to reliably affect recall. Some key influences include:

- **Anxiety**: more anxious patients seem to have better recall
- **Medical knowledge**: patients with greater knowledge have better recall
- **Primacy effect**: patients have better recall for the first information presented to them
- **Importance**: statements perceived by the patient to be important are recalled better
- **Volume of information**: when more information is presented, more is recalled but the percentage remembered is lower. (Broome and Llewelyn 1995)

The influences on memory described above, and other effects on recall, can be explained by looking at two theories of memory; the multistore model and levels of processing theory.

Anxiety

Anderson *et al.* (1979) found that higher levels of anxiety were associated with better recall. However, Bush and Osterweis (1978) found the reverse, suggesting that patient anxiety impaired the ability to learn new information (such as treatment regimens, explanations for their condition or appointment times).

Several psychological theories could account for these differences. Treisman (1964) suggested that our attention is directed towards pertinent information. Since attending to information is essential if we are to remember, it would be predicted that, for patients who are most anxious, information about their condition has greater pertinence so is more likely to be attended to and therefore has a higher probability of being recalled.

Once attended to, advice must then be retained and retrieved in order to be followed. Tulving (1974) suggested that we are better at retrieving stored information when we are in the same psychological state at the time of recall as we were during learning because our condition can act as a cue. This is called state dependency. Highly anxious patients are likely to remain so; therefore their state can provide a cue for recall, whereas less anxious patients may experience a wider range of emotions so are less likely to consistently provide state-dependent cues for recall.

Freud (1901) proposed repression as an explanation for forgetting when it is associated with particularly traumatic experiences. Repressed information is blocked from consciousness so cannot be recalled. This could account for reduced recall in patients who have been traumatised by finding out they have a serious condition about which they were unaware, or those who are in great pain or distress.

Existing medical knowledge

In an experimental study, Brown and Park (2002) found – in contrast to received wisdom – that both younger and older participants learned more information about an unfamiliar disease than a familiar one. They concluded that health care professionals should consider that patients may have difficulty recalling new information about familiar diseases. This may be accounted for, at least in part, because new information about a condition may contradict existing knowledge. Rice and Okun (1994) found that medical information that conflicted with patients' existing beliefs was recalled less accurately than information that did not. Such findings are supported by psychological evidence relating to interference in memory.

Forgetting triggered by new information may be initiated in two ways. Proactive inhibition, as seen in these examples, arises when we have to learn new facts but old ones 'get in the way'. We experience this when we persist in writing last year's date on cheques well into February or answer the telephone in our new house with the old phone number. In contrast, new memories can also 'overwrite' and obliterate old ones. When we learn a new PIN number or car registration, we experience difficulty recalling the previous one, a process called retroactive inhibition.

Perceived importance of information

As we discussed on page 98, according to Treisman's model of attention, patients are more likely to attend to and therefore recall information that they perceive to be pertinent to them. So, in order to increase adherence, we should ensure that patients perceive that the advice given is important for them as individuals. In Chapter 2, we considered the predictions of the Health Belief Model (page 58). This suggests that patients also recognise information as important for them if they believe themselves to be at risk, either because they are vulnerable or because their condition is serious. In the absence of these beliefs an individual would not attribute importance to advice given, so the model suggests that they would be unlikely to adhere.

The multistore model of memory

The multistore model of memory (Atkinson and Shiffrin 1968) suggests that incoming information is passed through three memory stores, each holding information for longer than the last. The first, the short-term sensory store (STSS), lasts only a matter of seconds, passing some but not all of its information on. If we fail to pay attention to information it will be lost at this stage. The remaining information is passed on the short-term memory (STM). This store last for about 30 seconds, although by repetition or **rehearsal** information can be kept in STM for longer. It is this same process of rehearsal that results in the transfer of information to the most permanent store, the long-term memory (LTM).

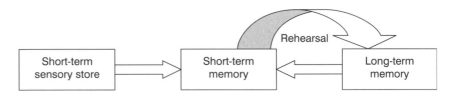

The multistore model of memory

Rehearsal

If we do not have the opportunity to 'play the information over' in our minds, then new information will not be transferred from STM to LTM and will be forgotten. Patients may find that they need to ask health professionals to repeat instructions or explanations in order to remember. Staff and patients may find this frustrating but rehearsal is one way to improve recall. MacKinnon and Fenaughty (1993) found that users of cigarettes, smokeless tobacco products and alcohol, who had therefore experienced greater exposure to health warnings so had had more opportunity to rehearse these messages, demonstrated better recall for the content of such labels than non-users.

Displacement

Our short-term memory has a limited capacity. We can only store about seven items at a time; any more than this and new information starts to push older information out of STM before it has been transferred to LTM. This cause of forgetting is called **displacement**. If a health care professional answers a patient's question but then immediately follows this with a question themselves without giving the patient the opportunity to rehearse the information, the original answer may be displaced and forgotten.

So, if patients receive too many pieces of information at one time, they may begin to 'lose' some of the items. An item or 'chunk' is a

Keywords

Rehearsal
Internal repetition that helps to transfer information from short-term to long-term memory

Keywords

Displacement
Forgetting from short-term memory that occurs because the capacity of STM is limited to about seven 'chunks' of information. If more than seven items arrive so quickly that they cannot be transferred to LTM, the newest items will push old ones out of STM

single piece of information. To a patient, for whom medical information is novel, each fact will be a separate chunk occupying a space in STM. This makes the material harder to remember for patients than it is for experienced professionals.

The process of displacement can account for the primacy effect, the tendency to have better recall for the earliest items presented. Murdock (1962) conducted an experiment in which participants heard a list of words then had to recall words from different parts of the list. They were best at remembering items from the beginning (the primacy effect) and the end (called the recency effect). Their recall for items from the middle of the list was poor. The primacy effect arises because the early items are rehearsed and transferred from STM to LTM. Patients therefore have good recall for the earliest information they are given (Ley 1972, 1982). Later items may be displaced by additional incoming information. More recently, Andrews and Carroll (1998) have also found a marked primacy effect in the memory for medical information.

It may be difficult for practitioners to see why patients have difficulty. As we saw in Chapter 1, health care practitioners have a 'register' or professional language which, when used inappropriately with less informed patients, is perceived as unintelligible jargon. Familiarity with words or ideas enables you to make bigger 'chunks'. When you first began to learn about psychology you probably had to spell the word letter by letter or in two 'sections' or chunks; now – hopefully – you can write the whole word without thinking. It has become a single chunk that takes up correspondingly less space in STM.

> ## Over to you
>
> To give yourself an idea of the patient's experience, try this task. If you can, work in pairs using lists written by your partner. Write out two sets of complex words, for example drug names, unusual conditions or terms relating to a specialist area. One set should consist of unfamiliar words, the other equally long familiar ones and each set should be 20 words long. Muddle the words from the two sets together to make a single list (also retain the original sets). If you are working alone, put the list out of sight for a couple of days. Now arm yourself with a blank sheet of paper and a pen. Allow 30 seconds to learn the list then cover it up. Now count backwards in threes from 100 to zero. As soon as you have finished, try to write down as many of the words as you can. Which original set did you recall more of? Why?

So, patients have two problems relating to displacement. First, information may be presented very quickly, so they don't have time to rehearse ideas and transfer them to LTM before they are displaced by later information. Second, because the concepts and terms are unfamiliar they cannot chunk the information so their STM fills up more quickly and displacement is more likely to occur.

Key points | **Top tips**

- Information must be rehearsed in order to be transferred from short-term memory to long-term memory, otherwise it will be forgotten
- If more than approximately seven chunks of information are presented quickly, the early ones will be displaced and forgotten rather than transferred to long-term memory.

The levels of processing theory of memory

Keywords

Semantic processing
The use of information based on its meaning that results, according to levels of processing theory, in good recall

Craik and Lockhart (1972) proposed the levels of processing theory of memory. This suggests that our memory consists of only one store but that information within it may be retained in different ways. According to Craik and Lockhart, by dealing with or 'processing' information more deeply, we are more likely to remember it. Deep or **semantic processing** occurs when we think about the meaning of information, for example, when we are trying to understand how an organ of the body works or why one course of treatment is better than another. There are three levels of processing:

- Structural processing relies only on superficial aspects, such as what an item looks like. For example, a patient may know the shape of the tablets they take or the colour of the box, or remember that following the red line through the hospital will get them to the X-ray department and the green line to the plaster room. It is the shallowest level of processing and results in the poorest recall.

- Phonemic processing uses information about the sound of the item to be remembered, for example if it sounds like another word or whether items rhyme. Children using preventer and reliever inhalers might remember 'use **br**own after **br**eakfast, keep **blue** with **you**'. It results in better recall than structural processing because it is deeper.

- Semantic processing deals with the meaning of information. It is the deepest level of processing and results in the best recall.

When patients are given information they need to be able to process it deeply in order to remember it but this may not be possible if they do not understand the concepts being discussed. Patients may be unfamiliar with bodily processes such as circulation so find the action of vasodilators or antihypertensives hard to comprehend. It is important therefore to ensure that patients receive sufficient explanation and that it is presented in an accessible way.

> ### Over to you
>
> Write a list of some of the terms and ideas that you have been taught in lectures over the last term or semester. Try to write a brief definition or summary of each. Put a tick beside those you feel confident that you understood at the time and a cross by those that were a little murky. Compare your definitions to those you were given on your course. Levels of processing theory would predict that the accuracy of your recall for those you put a tick beside would be much better than those with a cross. Why?

The effect of jargon

As we saw on page 14, using jargon can affect a patient's ability to remember information because a lack of understanding means that we cannot 'chunk' the items to be remembered. Levels of processing theory identifies another problem – using jargon can act as a barrier to deep processing. If patients are prevented from understanding what is meant by descriptions of symptoms or explanations of treatments because the terms being used are unfamiliar, they can only process the simple – structural or phonemic – aspects of the words (what they look and sound like). This shallow processing leads to poor recall of the information.

> ### Reflective activity
>
> Next time you have the opportunity to observe an experienced practitioner interacting with a patient, listen to what they are saying. Identify examples of:
> - Presenting too much information or saying it too quickly so that the patient could experience displacement
> - Pausing to give the patient time to 'absorb' the information
> - Using technical terms and concepts that the patient could find hard to understand and therefore 'chunk'
> - Explaining terms or using non-technical alternatives.

Key points Top tips

Understanding:

● Many patients do not understand the information they are given so cannot adhere to it

● Better understanding is not always related to better adherence

Satisfaction:

● Satisfied patients tend to have better adherence but this in turn may be affected by both memory and understanding

● Satisfaction and effective communication are related for clinicians too

Memory:

● Patients cannot adhere to information they cannot remember

● Different kinds of information are recalled differently – advice about medication may be better remembered than that about exercise or diet

● Many factors – repetition, too much information, use of jargon, unfamiliar or already familiar ideas and understanding – affect patients' ability to recall advice

---

Illness, treatment and adherence

Factors relating to the individual's condition, such as its severity, whether they are in pain and the nature of the treatment, are also important in explaining variability in adherence.

Seriousness of the illness and patient pain

It is a surprising finding that a patient who, according to their doctor, has a serious illness is no more likely to adhere to advice than one with a minor complaint. In fact, Haynes (1979) observed that 'not a single study has found that increasing severity of symptoms encourages compliance' (page 51). A typical finding, from Vincent (1971), showed that more than half the glaucoma patients studied did not follow simple advice to use eye drops and even when their vision deteriorated to extent that they were legally blind in one eye the compliance rate was still below 60%. In contrast, both the severity of the illness, as perceived by the patient, and their experience of pain predicted adherence (Becker and Maiman 1980, Becker 1979).

The parallel response model

One explanation for these observations is offered by Leventhal's parallel response model (Leventhal 1970). This suggests that, in a situation perceived to be dangerous, as could be the case with a serious illness, the individual appraises the threat in two independent ways:

- **Danger control**: motivation that results in adaptive behaviour to reduce the danger, such as following health advice, in order to overcome fear

- **Fear control**: motivation directed towards reducing fear, such as ignoring symptoms and advice and engaging in maladaptive behaviours like drinking that may offer comfort in the short term.

If a patient is more highly motivated to control their fear than the danger, perhaps because they have little faith in the efficacy of treatment or are very afraid (as may arise in the case with diagnosis of a serious illness), Leventhal's model suggests that they are unlikely to adhere to advice. The model can therefore explain the lack of relationship between severity of illness and adherence.

media watch   **Stop or you won't see your children grow up**

The hospital specialist looked serious. 'If you don't stop smoking . . . you won't live to see your children grow up.'

Janice Mathews was shocked. She had been coming to the hospital because of breathlessness and chest problems. . . . [She] had started smoking at the age of 12 and now had a 20- to 30-a-day habit. Her three children . . . often begged her to quit and she had tried, unsuccessfully . . . .

Sadly, smoking had permanently damaged her lungs and Janice developed COPD – chronic obstructive pulmonary disease. She needed two major lung reduction operations. These meant that she could use what lung she had left, better. . . .

She needs oxygen through a nasal tube 24 hours a day. Without it she cannot walk or talk.

As it is, she can't get dressed, wash her hair or get into bed without help. She can't cook, climb the stairs or do anything physical. . . .

You may have seen Janice in a television advert for the *Don't Give Up Giving Up* campaign. She agreed to be filmed to encourage others to quit smoking. She says . . . 'When I finally gave up smoking I was annoyed how easy I found it – the patches did it for me in the end. I wished I'd stopped a lot sooner, but I kept saying "I'll give up next month".'

Edited from *Take a Break*, 15 January 2004, pages 36–37.

When treatment is unpleasant: side effects and time

Another surprising finding is that, contrary to logic, patients are as likely to be compliant when medication is unpleasant as when there are no side effects (Masur 1981). However, in some cases, side effects could be sufficient to induce rational non-adherence. For example, Bulpitt *et al.* (1989) found that medication for hypertension that was successful in reducing symptoms such as headaches and depression also had side effects resulting in sexual difficulties such as impotence. As we saw on page 92, the behavioural model can account for non-adherence when undesirable side effects act as punishers.

Patients are, however, less likely to comply when treatment is prolonged. Haynes (1976) found that compliance rates fell as treatment duration increased – patients are more likely to drop out from longer treatment programmes than shorter ones. This finding may alternatively be attributable to the nature of different conditions. Those requiring sustained attention, such as high blood pressure, may have fewer symptoms to trigger compliance. Patients may therefore fail to adhere to treatment in the absence of evidence of their own illness rather than because the duration of treatment is lengthy.

DiMatteo and DiNicola (1982) reported that, while 70–80% of patients adhered to short-term medication regimens, less than 60% stuck to preventative programmes and even fewer – not even 50% – adhered to medical advice that required lifestyle changes. This illustrates another issue. Treatment for acute conditions, such as medication, requires little change to routine or habits so is relatively easy to adhere to. Following advice for the management of chronic conditions will more often require a significant lifestyle change, in diet, exercise or habits such as smoking. To consistently adhere to such recommendations demands a significantly greater effort on the part of the patient.

The complexity of treatment

Cramer *et al.* (1989) found that as treatment becomes more complex (when more drug doses must be taken each day) adherence falls:

- One daily dose: 88% adherence
- Three daily doses: 77% adherence
- Four daily doses: 39% adherence.

This pattern may arise because for one, two or three daily doses patients can identify an existing pattern to follow ('on waking', 'morning and night' or 'after meals'). This breaks down for a regime requiring four daily doses.

Pharmacist

Professionally speaking . . .

Helping patients to adhere – the role of the pharmacist

Do people ask for advice from your pharmacy?
A wide range of advice is sought from pharmacies from a wide range of people, health professionals and the public. Advice is requested about prescription medicines, minor ailments, alternative as well as conventional medicines, life-style advice and health supplements, to name just a few. The nature of advice sought is different in hospital pharmacies from retail pharmacies, as there are more clinical questions in hospital settings.

Has the frequency of such questioning risen with the appearance of 'ask your pharmacist' advertising?
Questioning has increased since the campaign, although I have no idea of how much.

Do you think the information provided with medicines is suitable?
Labels and PILS (Patient information leaflets) are invaluable, but the verbal reinforcement of all issues is ideal. Counselling patients at the outset of medication and ongoing communication that gives practical advice increases compliance.

Do people ever return to ask questions and, if so, are they ones that could be answered by reading the leaflet enclosed with the medicine?
People often return or phone post-prescription, usually for reassurance, but also to clarify their interpretation of the information we give. They often just want confirmation that they are doing the right thing.

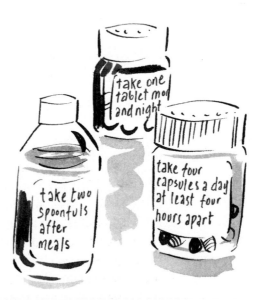

More complex treatment schedules are harder to follow and result in poorer adherence

Adherence and characteristics of the individual

Are some people more likely to comply than others? This section looks at a range of factors that affect the incidence of adherence in different individuals.

Gender and age

In some respects, men and women are equally compliant, for example in taking medication for hypertension (Monane *et al.* 1996). Similarly, Lynch *et al.* (1992) found that men and women with high levels of blood cholesterol were equally likely to stick to an exercise programme. However, some differences have been identified. Women are more likely to take medication for schizophrenia (Sellwood and Tarrier 1994) and to follow dietary advice about the consumption of fruit and vegetables (Laforge *et al.* 1994).

With regard to the age of patients, there are few consistencies in the results of studies. Patients of different ages appear to be more compliant in different situations. The overall findings suggest that factors other than age are probably more important predictors of compliance.

Social support: family and friends

Individuals living with a spouse or relative (Lorenc and Branthwaite 1993) or with close social relationships (Doherty *et al.* 1983) are, in general, more likely to adhere to medical advice than isolated people. For example, Bovbjerg *et al.* (1995) found that men whose wives were supportive were more likely to stick to a prescribed change in diet than those whose families were unsupportive. Similarly, Sherbourne *et al.* (1992) reported that adherence to advice about managing diabetes was better in individuals who had more social support. In a study that manipulated levels of support, Tanner and Feldman (1997) found that individuals whose significant other (e.g. partner) received supportive counselling were more likely to attend subsequent appointments.

It is unsurprising, therefore, to find that lack of social support impacts negatively on adherence. For example, Miller-Johnson *et al.* (1994) found that a key factor in non-adherence is increased conflict within a family. However, Sherwood (1983) found that haemodialysis patients were most likely to comply if their families were neither too over- nor under-involved emotionally. This suggests that social support is vital but that a measure of independence may also be important.

Personality and beliefs

As with findings about age and adherence, there is little evidence for links between adherence and personality in the general population. In fact, some studies have clearly demonstrated that the same individual will show different levels of compliance in differing situations (Lutz *et al.* 1983, Orme and Binik 1989). However, some specific groups do demonstrate differences. Individuals with obsessive-compulsive disorder (OCD) are, perhaps unsurprisingly, more compliant. Kabat-Zin and Chapman-Waldrop (1988) found that people with high scores on an OCD scale were more likely to stick to an 8-week stress-reduction programme than those with low scores.

Conversely, the results of one study suggested that some identifiable individuals are less likely to adhere to medical advice. Christensen *et al.* (1997) used a scale of cynical hostility (which measures personality characteristics such as suspiciousness, anger and resentfulness) to assess haemodialysis patients. Those with high scores were less likely to adhere to advice on diet and medication. Lack of adherence is also characteristic of individuals with avoidance-based coping mechanisms (Sherbourne *et al.* 1992). Avoidant individuals employ strategies such as 'something will turn up' and 'it might simply disappear' (see also external locus of control, page 111).

Unlike stable personality traits, some temporary changes in an individual's emotional state do appear to be linked to increased or reduced compliance. Optimistic patients are more likely follow treatment advice (Leedham *et al.* 1995) whereas depressed patients are less likely to (Carney *et al.* 1995). Similarly, Cipher *et al.* (2002) investigated compliance in patients suffering chronic pain. They found that those who suppressed negative emotions (such as anger) showed greater adherence to treatment whereas those with amplified negative emotions were less compliant.

In contrast to the relative absence of evidence for the effects of personality on adherence, personal beliefs do seem to be important. According to the health belief model (page 58), patients are more likely to adhere to advice when they:

- **Perceive themselves to be vulnerable**: e.g. a woman recognising that breast cancer could run in her own family so she should follow advice to attend screening
- **Perceive their condition to be serious**: e.g. having known several women who have died of cervical cancer encouraging a woman to respond to an invitation to have a smear test

- **Believe that their health will benefit from adherence**: e.g. an asthmatic who knows that using their preventer will improve their breathing is more likely to follow guidance to do so
- **Perceive few barriers to adherence**: e.g. a patient who believes that a dietary programme can be maintained so is more likely to stick to it
- **Have their behaviour prompted by a cue to action**: e.g. receiving a reminder to attend an appointment may encourage an individual to go for a dental check-up.

An example of these factors in action comes from Glasgow *et al.* (1986), who demonstrated that adolescents with diabetes were less likely to adhere to advice when they perceived the barriers to be significant. Meichenbaum and Turk (1987) observe that people are less likely to follow advice when they judge that barriers (such as side effects) exceed possible benefits (such as long-term health). This perception may be enhanced by an awareness of the reality that conscientious adherence can lead to more side effects (Kaplan and Simon 1990).

The theory of planned behaviour (page 64) suggests that patients are more likely to adhere to advice when:

- They have a positive attitude towards the behaviour required by compliance
- The subjective norms support compliance
- They therefore perceive themselves to be in control of their behaviour
- They intend to comply with the advice.

Again, evidence supports this idea. For example, Horne and Weinman (2002) investigated adherence to preventer medication by asthmatics. They found that individuals who had doubts about the necessity of the medication and concerns about its side effects (indicating a negative attitude towards compliance) were less likely to adhere.

Finally, we explore the ideas of self-efficacy and locus of control. Self-efficacy is an individual's confidence in their own ability to perform a behaviour. When a patient is confident that they can comply with advice, they are more likely to do so. For example, an asthmatic patient who believes they are able to use their inhaler competently is more likely to adhere to advice about usage than an individual who does not feel they can use it successfully. Research supports this prediction. Tedesco *et al.* (1991) found that self-efficacy was a good predictor of the likelihood that adults would brush and floss their teeth and McAuley (1993) reported that individuals with high self-efficacy were more likely to have stuck to an aerobic exercise programme for 4 months.

Locus of control refers to whether the individual believes that they are responsible for their own health outcomes (internal locus of control) or that their health is governed by factors beyond their control (external locus of control). Individuals with a high internal locus of control feel that they have personal choice so are more likely to follow advice because this enables them to exert their control over the situation. For example, Koski-Jannes (1994) found that those participants on an abstinence programme for alcoholics who had a strong internal locus of control were more likely to maintain their abstinence. However, self-determination does not guarantee adherence. Even when people choose to book an appointment with their doctor themselves they do not necessarily attend – Deyo and Inui (1980) estimated that between 15% and 60% of appointments are missed.

media watch 'I get a lot more kissing now I've quit'

I started smoking when I was still at school. By the time I was in my twenties pretty much all of my friends smoked. I sometimes thought about giving up, but I was convinced that if I quit I'd put on weight.

Then, just over a year ago, I went on a week's holiday to Turkey with four of my girlfriends. Two of them didn't smoke, one had just successfully given up using the NHS Smoking Helpline (0800 1690169) and the fourth had been in touch with her local NHS Stop Smoking Service and was waiting for her first meeting. That left just me.

I hadn't really been feeling particularly happy with myself and my habit. I woke up with a cough every morning and I was forever thinking about when I could have my next drag – to the point that whenever I was going on train or plane journeys my main thought was 'how am I going to manage without a cigarette?' I hated the fact that cigarettes controlled me so much.

It also dawned on me that going to the gym to keep fit and well was pretty pointless if I was then reaching for a fag straight away – it was as if I was going forwards and backwards at the same time.

As soon as I got back from holiday I rang the Helpline and enrolled with my local NHS Stop Smoking Service. This meant going along to weekly group counselling sessions.

I decided to choose 20 January last year as a quit date. January seemed the perfect month to make a decision which was going to affect the rest of my life, but I wanted to wait until after the New Year festivities to make it easier on myself.

The key was preparation. I was encouraged to think about the times I smoked and why, and what I could do instead of having a cigarette. I wasn't sure about going to a meeting with a bunch of people I didn't really know, but the group turned out to be really supportive. Everybody contributed something different.

I picked up lots of good ideas. For instance, someone told me to put a bendy straw in a bottle of water and keep it by the computer or the phone. Then every time I felt the urge to light up, I was to hold the straw like a cigarette and drink.

continued

It was a lot easier to give up cigarettes than I'd thought it would be, although I had one bad moment at a wedding when a friend started to smoke. Suddenly I really wanted a cigarette. My partner Pete was wonderful, though. He told me I'd done really well and reminded me how far I'd come. So I managed to resist temptation – and afterwards I felt very pleased with myself.

I've been a non-smoker for almost a year now. I haven't put on any weight, despite my fears, as I've made a conscious effort to eat really healthily. I sleep much better and I don't wake up with a racking, chesty cough.

My flat doesn't smell, nor do my hair or clothes. And I get a lot more kissing now.

Rachel Jayne Clarke

From *Take a Break*, 15 January 2004, pages 36–37.

Over to you

Despite considerable medical advice recommending that smokers give up, many continue to smoke. Consider the article above in the light of the ideas raised in the chapter so far – how much of Rachel's reluctance to quit and subsequent success can you explain?

The effect of culture

In a multicultural society, health professionals will encounter individuals from a range of different cultures. Cultural beliefs may represent an additional reason for some instances of non-adherence, for example if traditional treatments for or expectations about illness conflict with recommendations from health care practitioners. Harwood (1971) provides an example from the study of a Puerto Rican population in New York. Lay Puerto Rican health beliefs divide diseases, foods and treatments into 'hot' and 'cold' domains and cultural expectations of medication are that 'cold' illnesses should be countered with 'hot' medication and *vice versa*. So if penicillin (a 'hot' drug) were prescribed for a 'cold' condition such as rheumatic heart disease, this would be adhered to but as a treatment for 'hot' illness, such as diarrhoea or constipation, it would be ignored. As a consequence, some non-adherence arises when pharmacological advice and cultural beliefs conflict.

Health practitioner behaviour and adherence

Just as differences between patients affect adherence, so do the characteristics of different health care practitioners. Factors such as their communication skills, communication style, competence and gender can each affect adherence by the patient.

Communication skills

As we discussed in Chapter 1, effective communication plays a key role in good health care and is therefore important to adherence. DiMatteo *et al.* (1986) compared doctors' sensitivity to non-verbal cues (as assessed by their accuracy in understanding audiotaped examples) and the frequency with which their patients cancelled and failed to reschedule appointments. They found that those doctors who were most attuned to the cues of others had more reliable patients.

In speaking to patients, doctors focus on the task of diagnosis; asking questions and obtaining sufficient information to come to a conclusion about their diagnosis or proposed treatment. Doctors may therefore be selective in the aspects of a patient's answers to which they respond. A patient, however, may be concerned about one particular symptom that has little bearing on the diagnosis, so is ignored. As a consequence, the patient may conclude that the doctor is not listening to them or is not concerned, and therefore may feel unsatisfied with their treatment. This dissatisfaction can lead to reduced compliance (see page 96). Furthermore, patients may cease to attend to the doctor's instructions, further reducing the possibility of compliance (see page 99).

Elsewhere we have discussed various roles for emotion – its impact on patients' memory (page 97) and on communication. For example, we have discussed the benefits of a more emotionally focused communication style. However, emotionality in the health care context is not always beneficial. Evidence from a study conducted by Rorer *et al.* (1988) suggests that emotionally toned information, whether it is positive or negative, is less likely to result in compliance. Patients on haemodialysis were most likely to adhere to instructions when the nurse–patient relationship was maintained with emotionally neutral responses.

Practitioner characteristics: competence, communication style and gender

Patients are more likely to adhere to recommendations if they have confidence in the competence of the health care practitioner (Gilbar 1989). Similarly, DiNicola and DiMatteo (1984) found that doctors perceived to be friendly and caring, characteristic of a patient-focused approach (see page 35), were more likely to gain compliance from their patients, and DiMatteo *et al.* (1994) reported that patients were more likely to adhere to advice if their doctor was willing to answer all their questions, even when this took a long time – typical of a patient-centred approach. In contrast, authoritarian health practitioners, whose approach is doctor-focused (see page 9) and who tend to exclude the patient from the decision making process, are less likely to have compliant patients (Gastorf and Galanos 1983). We might predict, therefore, that women doctors, who tend to employ a more patient-focused approach (see page 35), would have more compliant patients.

Reflective activity

Consider the list of reasons for non-adherence listed below and try to think of examples you have encountered that would fit into as many categories as you can. Remember, an individual may have several reasons not to adhere.

- Failing to attend to instructions
- Being unable to understand instructions
- Being unable to remember instructions
  - Anxiety
  - Medical knowledge
  - Primacy effect
  - Importance
  - Volume of information
  - No opportunity for rehearsal
  - Displacement
- Feeling unsatisfied with the health practitioner
- Seriousness of the illness
- Patient pain
- Patient fear
- Side effects of treatment
- Duration of treatment
- Complexity of treatment
- Gender of patient
- Age of patient
- Social support
- Personality of patient
- Beliefs of patient
- Culture of patient
- Confidence in practitioner
- Communication skills of practitioner
- Communication style of practitioner
- Gender of practitioner.

Key points | Top tips

- The patient's perception of their pain, but not the clinician's, increases adherence
- Side effects, time taken to follow advice and the complexity of treatment negatively impact on adherence
- Patient gender and age show few reliable effects on adherence whereas greater adherence is associated with social support and personality factors such as obsessive-compulsive disorder
- Models that predict health behaviour suggest factors that are likely to affect adherence – such as the influence of perceived barriers, self-belief and locus of control – and evidence supports these
- Cultural beliefs can act to increase or decrease adherence
- Health practitioner characteristics, such as competence and communication style, can increase adherence.

Improving compliance with medical information

Research into the rates of adherence carries with it the implicit assumption that, for the patient, adhering to medical advice will be beneficial. Is this assumption also supported by research?

Little investigation has been carried out but that which has actually suggests that the benefits may be slight or non-existent. Patients may be no worse off for having ignored advice. In fact, Inui *et al.* (1981) suggested that, based on evidence from pill counts, 40% of well-controlled hypertensives were in fact non-adherent. This implies that at least some advice may be unnecessary and – at least for some patients, some of the time – non-adherence does not have significant negative consequences.

In fact, a 4-year study conducted by Hays *et al.* (1994) found few if any benefits from adherence. They investigated adherence in 2125 patients from four groups (people with diabetes, hypertension, congestive heart failure and recent myocardial infarction). Adherence was measured as the extent to which the patients followed advice given – for example eating a low-salt diet. Each patient's adherence was compared to health outcomes, assessed using measures such as limitations of role due to physical or emotional problems, pain, fatigue and physical functioning. The researchers' findings showed that – for most patients – the association between improved health and good adherence was little above chance and that, for insulin-dependent diabetic patients and those who were depressed, adherence was related to poorer physical health.

In addition to the apparent absence of evidence for the value of adherence, some doubt has been cast on the cause of improved health when adherence is good. Horowitz and Horowitz (1993) report that several studies have demonstrated improved health in patients who adhere to advice on taking medication compared to non-adherers, even when the drug they are taking is a placebo.

There are clearly some issues over the value of adherence. Nevertheless, we can only expect patients to comply at all if certain criteria are met, such as that we ensure patients understand, believe and remember the messages they have been given. The following sections are devoted to exploring how aspects of patient care can be changed to improve the rate of adherence to medical advice.

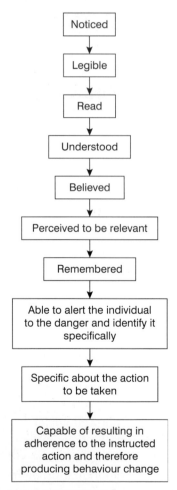

Conditions for a health message to be effective

In the following sections we will explore how we can use psychological knowledge to improve adherence at various stages along the route identified by Ley and Llewelyn (1995).

Improving patient attention to and understanding of medical information

Improving attention

In order for patients to comply, they must be aware of and be able to hear, or see and read, the message intended for them. Some ways to ensure that this is achieved are suggested in the box below.

Getting the message noticed

- Verbal warnings e.g. 'Danger' Hazard' or 'Caution'
- Using colour, bold, size, fonts, borders, prominent position
- Graphic symbols
- Attention-raising gimmicks e.g. flip books for putting on condoms
- Making the message legible or audible – in print, use good contrast, size and spacing to ensure readability and avoid writing text in capitals

Improving understanding

Ley and Llewelyn (1995) have identified two aspects of spoken communication that help to improve patient understanding, so are implicated in adherence:

- Important points should be stressed – according to Ley (1972) this increases recall by 15%
- Information should be simplified, using shorter words and sentences – Bradshaw *et al.* (1975) report that this increased recall by 13%

In addition to suggesting ways to increase adherence by improving spoken communication, Ley and Llewelyn (1995) also recommended the use of written communication. There are several reasons for this:

- Even when good practice in spoken communication is evident, non-compliance may still be a problem (Ley 1988)
- The content of written material can be designed to maximise understandability and memorability
- Written material can be used as a source of reference for patients
- Patients want printed information – e.g. Gibbs *et al.* (1990) found that 97% of a sample of British patients would like to receive written information about their medication.

Of course, just because patients demonstrate a desire for written material does not mean that supplying it will necessarily lead to improved adherence. The information must still be read, understood and followed. From a series of studies conducted in Britain, Gibbs *et al.* (1987) have reported that 88% of 117 patients taking penicillin or non-steroidal anti-inflammatory drugs (NSAIDs) read leaflets about their drugs and 97% of a sample of 349 patients taking NSAIDs, beta-adrenoceptor antagonists or inhaled bronchodilators claimed to have read their leaflets (Gibbs *et al.* 1989). These figures are encouragingly high. Estimates from Ley (1988) for US samples have found variable percentages of patients claiming to have read leaflets about their medication (49–97%) but fewer (22–57%) kept the leaflets and referred to them.

The understandability of printed medical information has also been investigated and most studies show that this information is too difficult for most people to comprehend. In a summary comparing the results of a range of studies, Ley and Llewelyn (1995) estimated that 27% of leaflets demanded such an advanced level of reading that 69% of the population would not understand them! This percentage rises to 83% for patients over 65 years of age required to understand leaflets of the same degree of difficulty. This summary was based on the findings of studies predominantly conducted in the 1970s, but the trend continues. For example, Richwald *et al.* (1988) found that instructions for condom use were too complex for their intended audience.

Over to you

Find two medicines that you or your family use and study the containers and leaflets. Read them carefully and decide which of the recommendations discussed above have been employed. Identify those that have not been followed and decide how the information or presentation could have been improved to maximise the likelihood of individuals adhering to the instructions and advice presented.

Finally, understanding may relate not only to understanding 'what' is required but also understanding 'how'. Skills training is designed to help patients to make appropriate judgements and perform required behaviours. McCulluch *et al.* (1983) used skills training to help patients with insulin-dependent diabetes to manage their diet correctly. The patients were offered menus from which they had to select appropriate foods and quantities, and received immediate feedback from a dietitian about their choices. Within 7 days a greater improvement was apparent in the dietary management of patients in the skills training group than in those receiving information or education only.

The effect of familiarity and cues to behaviour change

Even if patients have read warnings and understood them, they may still ignore them, especially if the message is very familiar. For example, research conducted at the Centre for Behavioural Research in Cancer (1992) found that individuals who had been smoking for longer were less likely to be able to recall warning messages on cigarette packets than were smokers who had acquired the habit more recently (although contrast this finding with that of MacKinnon and Fenaughty, page 100). One explanation for the apparent habituation to warning messages is offered by Breznitz (1984). According to Breznitz, the credibility of the message is reduced because the smoker has evidence that it is a 'false alarm' since they are able to smoke one, then progressively many cigarettes without any clear signal that the behaviour is damaging. Research conducted by Borland and Naccarella (1991) supports this view, as older smokers are less likely to attribute the cause of smoking-related illnesses to their habit.

Somewhat surprisingly, not even actual alarms such as accidents or injuries seem to act as effective cues to change behaviour. For example, Bragg (1973) found that seatbelt use was not affected by the occurrence of injuries in car accidents (contrast this finding with the evidence for the importance of cues to action according to the health belief model, page 64).

Improving patients' memory for medical information

In order to recall information, it must be attended to and, preferably understood, so attempts to make material more obvious or comprehensible will also improve memory for that information. In addition, based on the research discussed on pages 96–97, the following recommendations can be made that would specifically improve the likelihood of patients remembering information presented to them about health matters.

- Present information in small amounts (to enable chunking in STM)
- Ensure information can be understood (to allow deep processing to occur)
- Present key information first (so that the primacy effect ensures that it is transferred to LTM) – Ley (1972) showed that this improved recall by 36%
- Repeat key information (to improve rehearsal and transfer to LTM) – Ley (1979) and Bertakis (1977) showed that repetition increased recall and satisfaction

- Present information sufficiently slowly, or with gaps, to avoid displacement and do not ask questions immediately after providing information.

Houts *et al.* (1998) found that the provision of cues in the form of pictographs helped to improve recall for spoken medical instructions. The participants, students from a remedial reading class, were tested on their ability to remember a list of 38 instructions for managing fever and 50 for managing a sore mouth. They recalled only 14% of the verbal instructions without any cues but 85% when assisted by the visual memory cues.

Encouraging patients to follow advice that they understand and remember

Even if we are able to provide information that patients can understand and recall, this will not automatically lead to adherence – they must take steps to actually follow that advice. For example, in patients with diabetes, improving understanding through education does not guarantee better control of blood glucose or reduce hospitalisation (Goodall and Halford 1991, Shillitoe 1988). The following sections consider ways to make acting on advice more likely.

Applying the behavioural model: reinforcing adherence

The processes of operant conditioning can be used to increase adherence. Patients can be provided with cues to trigger appropriate behaviours and such responses can be rewarded with positive reinforcement. Some reinforcers may be intrinsic, i.e. internal to the individual – such as feeling good about losing weight – whilst others are extrinsic, i.e. from an external source – such as praise from the health care professional. Hegel *et al.* (1992) successfully used positive reinforcers, shaping and self-management with haemodialysis patients to improve their adherence to dietary advice with requirements, for example, for reduced fluid intake and the control of protein, potassium and phosphorus consumption. They suggested that such strategies may be at least as effective at gaining adherence as cognitive approaches – and easier to implement.

Examples of cues for adherence:
- Postal, telephone or e-mail reminders for appointments
- Pill calendars or packets marked with days of the week
- Visual reminders such as hand-written notes.

Examples of positive reinforcers:

- Feeling fitter
- Money
- Stickers for children attending dental appointments.

The employment of a token economy is a way to ensure that positive reinforcers are contingent, and therefore effective. Patients are rewarded for adherence with tokens that can be exchanged later for desirable items or opportunities (such as watching television). Carney *et al.* (1983) found that a token economy programme was effective in improving control of blood glucose levels with three children with diabetes. They were awarded points for appropriate and accurate testing of blood glucose and received parental praise if they conducted the test within 10 minutes of the intended time.

The effectiveness of incentives can also be interpreted using the behavioural model. An incentive acts to 'suggest' the possibility of a reward, making the benefits of reinforcement desirable. Incentives can therefore act both as cues to trigger behaviour and as immediate (i.e. contingent) intrinsic reinforcers. An example of incentives in action would be the use of contracts between patients and health care professionals, for instance in gaining compliance from adolescents with insulin-dependent diabetes. The contract both provides a cue – a reminder of the action to be performed – and acts to generate a positive reinforcer – the satisfaction of knowing that you have fulfilled the contract.

Self-monitoring can also act as an incentive strategy, providing cues and intrinsic rewards. This has been used successfully by Wing *et al.* (1986) to assist patients with diabetes. The patients are equipped with the skills to monitor blood glucose levels accurately and use this information to regulate carefully with injections. They then reinforce themselves for improved blood glucose control and for adherence such as eating a good diet and taking exercise.

Enhancing personal relevance

One disadvantage of supplying patients with pre-printed material is that it must be general. This is problematic because patients are more likely to comply if the advice they are given is personally tailored so that they can see how it is relevant to them. This requires health care professionals to individualise instructions and to try to fit programmes (such as diet, exercise or taking of medication) into the individual's daily routine.

Pagoto *et al.* (2003) found that, in an intervention aimed at reducing the risk of skin cancer, beach goers were more likely to engage in sun protection if, in addition to education, they received personalised information about the risks of unprotected sun exposure.

Removing barriers to adherence

If the treatment programme can be kept short and simple, patients are more likely to adhere to it. For example, Haynes *et al.* (1987) found that patients were more likely to stick to a medication regimen if the doses were less frequent. The difficulty of organising or remembering is reduced, removing a barrier and increasing adherence.

Enhancing social support

Adherence can be improved by encouraging the patient's family or friends to become involved in understanding the treatment. Morisky (1983) found that hypertensive patients benefited from enhanced social support. Patients allocated to interventions involving home visits that aimed to increase social support were more likely to have survived 5 years later.

Encouraging self-efficacy

Individuals who believe that they can adhere are more likely to do so, so setting patients achievable goals should improve adherence. Borrelli and Mermelstein (1994) investigated self-efficacy and goal setting to success on a programme to help smokers to quit. They found that individuals who were more confident about being able to achieve the goal of giving up were more likely to succeed. Similarly, Kalichman *et al.* (2002) found that self-efficacy with regards to 'condom skills' predicted the use of condoms by male and female adolescents on a substance abuse treatment programme. However, Norman *et al.* (2003) found that, although parents of children with amblyopia (squint) who had higher self-efficacy were more motivated to comply with eye-patching, in fact, only perceived vulnerability and response costs (barriers) were significant predictors of adherence.

Key points Top tips

Adherence may be improved by strategies such as:

Improving attention:

- Make messages more noticeable and legible

Assisting understanding:

- Use simple, spoken instructions and stress important points
- Back this up with written information that is comprehensible
- Ensure that patients have the skills to follow the advice that has been given and recognise that it is relevant to them

Assisting memory:

- Present information slowly, in small amounts, most important points being made first and repeating advice

Assisting action:

- Identify and use cues, incentives and reinforcers for adherent behaviours
- Tailor advice for individuals to improve the likelihood of adherence
- Keep treatment programmes short and simple
- Encourage social support
- Set achievable goals to enhance self-efficacy.

Conclusions

Patients receiving medical treatment do not necessarily follow the advice they have been given. This may be the case even when they are told that they are seriously ill. Being afraid, having a complex medication regimen, suffering side effects or having to find time to make a change in lifestyle all tend to reduce adherence to medical advice. Patients who are in pain or who believe themselves to be very ill are more likely to adhere as are those who have good social support. Some factors, such as age, gender and personality, have few consistent effects on adherence. Health care practitioners themselves can also affect patients' adherence through their communication skills, communication style, competence and gender.

Non-adherence may be explained in a number of different ways: through the effects of factors that act as rewards (such as recovery) or punishment (such as side effects), or by a lack of understanding or recall by patients. Dissatisfied patients are also less likely to adhere to instructions. Health behaviour models additionally suggest that individuals who perceive few barriers to adherence, think that they will benefit, have cues to trigger the following of advice, have a positive attitude to treatment, believe that they are in control of their own behaviour and intend to comply with advice are more likely to do so.

The findings of research in this area provide a range of suggestions for ways to improve adherence to medical advice. Techniques aim to increase attention to, and memory and understanding of the advice given, enhance personal relevance of information, remove barriers to following the advice, increase social support and raise the patient's belief that they are able to adhere.

Reflective activity

Think back to an instance you have experienced or have read about in which a patient did not adhere to recommended advice. What explanations can you offer for their non-adherence? Consider why you believe that these particular reasons apply in this case. If you had been in a senior role, what might you have considered doing in order to improve their adherence and what reservations might you have had about your recommendations?

Rapid recap

Check your progress so far by working through each of the following questions.

1. What are the three factors that affect compliance to medical advice according to Ley's model?

2. Identify four factors that could affect a patient's ability to recall information they have been given.

3. Describe three ways that a health professional could improve adherence by changing the way spoken information is presented to patients.

If you have difficulty with more than one of the questions, read through the section again to refresh your understanding before moving on.

Key references

Other references are in the main reference list at the end of the book.

Leedham, B., Meyerowitz, B.E., Muirhead, J. and Frist, W.H. (1995) Positive expectations predict health after heart transplantation. *Health Psychology*, **13**: 74–79.

Ley, P. (1979) Memory for medical information. *British Journal of Social and Clinical Psychology*, **18**: 245–256.

Ley, P. and Llewelyn, S. (1995) Improving patients' understanding, recall, satisfaction and compliance. In: *Health Psychology: Processes and applications* (eds A. Broome and S. Llewelyn). Chapman & Hall, London, pp. 75–98.

Lorenc, L. and Branthwaite, A. (1993) Are older adults less compliant with prescribed medication than younger adults? *British Journal of Clinical Psychology*, **32**: 485–492.

MacKinnon, D.P. and Fenaughty, A.M. (1993) Substance use and memory for health warning labels. *Health Psychology*, **12**: 147–150.

Rice, G.E. and Okun, M.A. (1994) Older readers' processing of medical information that contradicts their beliefs. *Journal of Gerontology*, **49**: 119–128.

4

Stress

This chapter discusses biological and psychological explanations of stress, including the nervous, endocrine and immune systems and the roles of stressful life events and individuals' appraisal of the stressor. Being ill can be stressful and, conversely, the experience of stress can affect health. The links between stress and health are explored in a review of psychoneuroimmunology. Possible causes of stress are considered, including internal and external stressors and how they interact. In addition, a range of biological, social and psychological factors that affect the stress experienced by patients and staff is considered. Stress can affect social behaviour and performance as well as health and this has implications for the management of stress in patients and staff. Finally, strategies for coping with stress are discussed.

Learning outcomes

By the end of this chapter you should be able to:

- Define stress
- Discuss biological and psychological explanations of stress
- Describe research into the links between stress and health
- Describe sources of stressors for patients and health care professionals
- Identify biological, social and psychological factors that can increase an individual's experience of stress
- Identify ways in which stress can affect social behaviour and performance
- Describe and evaluate stress management strategies that could be used by patients and health care professionals.

The concept of stress

Stress is a reaction, both physical and psychological, to circumstances that are perceived to be negative and threatening to the individual. The elements of the situation that provoke such a response are called stressors. Some kinds of stimuli, under particular circumstances, may become stressful. Stressors could affect us in one of two ways:

- Physiologically by affecting body functioning such as altering pulse rate, blood pressure and the immune system or by changing hormone levels
- Psychologically through sensitivity changes in cognitive functioning and emotions such as fear or anger.

Some of these responses are, of course, adaptive; they help us to respond to potential dangers. However, they evolved to protect us when our environment was somewhat different from that in which we now live. The stress response that helped primitive humans avoid being eaten by fast-moving predators are of little help to a stressed patient awaiting surgery or an overworked sister faced with a ward filled beyond capacity. Neither would have much to gain by being able to run fast!

Factors involved in the explanation of stress

Stressors can be categorised as either internal (individual) or external (environmental). These two classes of stressor can also operate in combination.

Internal factors and stress

Some stressors are internal, that is they originate within us. The sensation of anxiety can arise without any obvious stimulus from the outside yet it can make us stressed. Although such feelings may be irrational and without an apparent cause they can nevertheless be very stressful. A range of thoughts and feelings may be stressful, worrying about things that may never happen such as fretting about not waking up from an anaesthetic or finding a malignant lump. Pain is also an internal source of stress; a nagging headache or chronic back pain could act as a stressor. Similarly, being ill or unable to sleep are internal experiences that can induce stress. An individual who lies in bed fretting about being tired the next morning because they cannot fall asleep is experiencing stress even though there may be no external trigger for their sleeplessness.

External factors and stress

In approaches that focus on external factors, stress is seen as something that happens to an individual rather than within them. Stress arises when levels of stressors such as the pressures of work become too high. Thus physical situations such as crowding or noise, and social situations such as missing a loved one, or being forced to engage with unpleasant or frightening people, is stressful. Being a new patient on a ward could therefore present external stressors. Life events theory (see page 135) identifies key occurrences such as changing jobs that are stressful.

The incidence of stress among health care professionals is known to be high (e.g. Borrill *et al.* 1998). Some reasons for this include lack of clarity about roles, conflict, excess work demands and lack of control over work. Such factors are external to the individual.

Interactional factors and stress

This approach suggests that stress arises from an interaction between the environment and the individual's response to it.

Importantly, it emphasises the psychological factors that allow some people to cope with more stressful environments than others.

Lazarus's appraisal model (see page 137) incorporates such an interaction. It suggests that the way an individual perceives and responds to a stimulus (i.e. copes) determines their experience of stress. When the individual judges their resources to be inadequate in comparison to their perception of the challenge, there are emotional and physiological responses and they feel stressed. This helps to explain why the relationship between a potential stressor and the stress an individual suffers is not a simple one. People may differ in the way they appraise, and therefore tackle, the demands of a situation as well as in their personal resources.

For example, one patient may experience a forthcoming procedure as something that will be unpleasant but that they can endure whereas another may anticipate that the consequences will be intolerable. Thus the second individual, but not the first, will experience stress as they appraise the situation to be difficult (or impossible) to cope with.

Theories of stress

Physiological explanations of stress

The physiological response to stress is mediated by two bodily systems. One, the autonomic nervous system, is composed of two approximately **antagonistic** sub-systems, the sympathetic and parasympathetic branches. The autonomic nervous system acts rapidly to stimulate physiological changes such as breathing and heart rate as well as affecting the second element, the **endocrine system**. The other, the endocrine system, provides a slower communication route through the body using **hormones** released in response to signals from nerves or from other glands.

Autonomic nervous system

In an emergency, the sympathetic branch of the autonomic nervous system responds quickly, preparing for 'fight or flight'. The sympathetic nervous system also sends impulses to the endocrine system, which responds by releasing hormones that enhance the preparation for action. This mechanism, which links the sympathetic nervous system to the **adrenal medulla**, is called the sympathetic adrenal medullary system (see page 129). Although the sympathetic response is very fast, allowing us to respond quickly to an emergency, its effects are short-lived.

Keywords

Antagonistic
Paired systems that work in opposition, such as parts of the nervous system that increase or decrease arousal

Endocrine system
Bodily communication route composed of glands releasing hormones that travel via the blood to target organs

Hormones
Chemicals released by endocrine glands into the blood stream that acts as a communication system in the body

Keywords

Adrenal medulla
The inner part of the adrenal glands, which releases the hormone adrenaline (epinephrine)

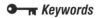

Keywords

Catecholamines

A group of neurotransmitters with a similar chemical structure to adrenaline that includes dopamine and noradrenaline (norepinephrine)

Adrenal cortex

The outer region of the adrenal glands, which releases corticosteroid hormones

Endocrine system

The effects of the endocrine system are slower but longer lasting. Adrenaline (epinephrine) is released from the adrenal medulla in response to stressors, as are related neurotransmitters (**catecholamines**) including noradrenaline (norepinephrine). This elevated level of catecholamines during stress may be responsible for some of the effects of stress on health such as hardening of the arteries. In addition, the **adrenal cortex** releases corticosteroid hormones. These processes are discussed further on page 130.

The general adaptation syndrome

Selye (1947) described the body's response to stress and began to explore the links between the nervous system, the endocrine system and illness. He induced stress in rats using stressors including heat and fatigue. The rats showed the same physiological responses regardless of the nature of the stressor; they had enlarged adrenal glands, shrunken lymph glands and stomach ulcers. Selye proposed that the body responded to any stressor by mobilising itself for action, a response he called the general adaptation syndrome. This response has evolved to help the individual to deal with emergency situations such as fleeing physical danger. Selye identified three phases to the body's response to stress through which an individual passes if a stressor persists over time:

● **Alarm reaction**: the body's mechanisms for dealing with danger are activated
● **Resistance stage**: the person struggles to cope with the stress and the body attempts to return to its previous physiological state
● **Exhaustion stage**: if the stressor persists and the body cannot return to its previous state, physical resources become depleted, eventually leading to collapse.

A great deal more is now known about the precise mechanisms controlling the response to stress than Selye first observed.

The sympathetic adrenal medullary system

In the initial response to a potentially threatening stimulus the sympathetic branch of the autonomic nervous system prepares the body quickly for action. The sympathetic response also causes the release of hormones, adrenaline and noradrenaline, from the adrenal medulla. The combined effect of the sympathetic adrenal medullary system ensures that the body is physically prepared to counter the environmental threat, for instance by fighting or fleeing.

The sympathetic adrenal medullary system therefore controls responses to acute (short-term) stressors. The effects of the sympathetic response, which resembles the action of adrenaline, is illustrated in the table below.

Over to you

Complete the table below, which lists some of the functions of the two parts of the autonomic nervous system.

Sympathetic effects	Parasympathetic effects
Increased heart rate	
Increased blood pressure	
Dry mouth	Maintenance of saliva production
Dilated pupils	
Dilated blood vessels in muscles	
Contracted blood vessels around digestive system	Blood supply to digestive system is increased to remove products of digestion
Increased sweating	
Increased breathing rate	

The hypothalamic–pituitary–adrenocortical axis

If the stressor is not removed the body responds differently, reducing levels of adrenaline and noradrenaline and increasing levels of three other hormones:

- Cortisol breaks down fatty tissue, releasing soluble fats and stimulating the release of glucose from the liver so that the muscles can obtain more energy from the blood
- Aldosterone increases blood pressure, maintaining the body ready for action
- Thyroxine increases the body's metabolic rate. This means that the stressed person can extract energy from food more quickly. Thyroxine also increases the rate at which food travels through the gut, allowing energy to be quickly obtained from the food currently in the gut.

The release of corticosteroids such as cortisol from the adrenal cortex is controlled by another hormone, adrenocorticotrophic hormone (ACTH) from the pituitary gland. ACTH is in turn secreted in response to the release of corticotrophin-releasing factor (CRF). CRF is a **peptide** released by the paraventricular nucleus, a region of the hypothalamus. Soendergaard and Theorell (2003) reported raised cortisol levels in refugees, particularly when they were

○━┓ Keywords

Peptide
A small protein

○━ᴨ *Keywords*

Aversive

Unpleasant (e.g. as a feature of the immediate environment)

experiencing distress in significant others (such as close friends or relatives) and excessive demands on everyday life.

Injection of CRF into the brain produces responses similar to those associated with **aversive** situations, supporting the belief that some aspects of the stress response are caused by CRF. For example, Swerdlow *et al.* (1986) found that CRF increased the startle response shown by rats to a loud noise. This link between the hypothalamus, the pituitary gland and the adrenal cortex is referred to as the hypothalamic–pituitary–adrenocortical axis and can trigger the release of corticosteroids to minor but unpredictable changes. If these are not threatening, the response diminishes as cortisol feeds back to the hypothalamus and pituitary gland to limit further releases of CRF and ACTH. If, however, the situation is sustained – in the case of a chronic stressor – the action of the hypothalamic–pituitary–adrenocortical axis is maintained by the forebrain.

Hypothalamic–pituitary–adrenal
(in response to a chronic stressor)

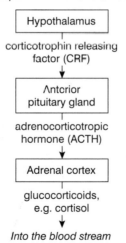

Sympathetic adrenal medullary system
(in response to an acute stressor)

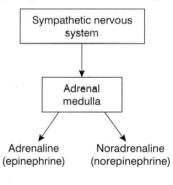

The effects of stressors

If the stressor is severe and prolonged, exhaustion may result. Examples of such stressors include being hunted, tortured or working in a high-demand profession such as nursing. Exhaustion occurs when the body's supplies of energy are used up. This may ultimately result in collapse and sometimes death. Furthermore, these systems are adapted to protect us from environmental stressors present in our evolutionary history – such as being chased by a sabre-toothed tiger – but we are now exposed to rather different problems, such as working shifts or talking to bereaved relatives.

One consequence of this biological endowment is that our coping strategies fail to deal effectively with the demands of modern living, causing chronic sympathetic adrenal medullary activation rather than leading to hypothalamic–pituitary–adrenocortical activity. The effects, such as prolonged elevation of pulse rate and blood pressure, put strain on the cardiovascular system with, perhaps, the consequence of increased levels of cardiovascular disorders. Where coping is less effective, for example because control is limited, another characteristic of modern living, hypothalamic–pituitary–adrenocortical activity will be triggered. Where such stressors are chronic, **immunosuppression** may result as corticosteroids such as cortisol affect immune functioning.

The two systems, the sympathetic adrenal medullary system and the hypothalamic–pituitary–adrenocortical axis have been represented here as independent although, in reality, they are not. The neurotransmitters noradrenaline and serotonin, natural endorphins and the hormone cortisol all act as intermediaries between the two systems.

Stress and the immune system

The immune system is a collection of structures and mechanisms that our bodies use to fight off disease. The lymphatic system consists of branching vessels that drain tissue fluid containing micro-organisms away from the cells of the body back into the blood. Various kinds of white blood cells called lymphocytes are responsible for different aspects of the immune response (Table 4.1). Changes in levels of these cells and their products (immunoglobulins) can be measured and related to levels of stress (Pitts and Phillips 1998).

○━🔑 Keywords

Immunosuppression
Reduced capacity of the body to fight disease due to deactivation of the immune response

---

Table 4.1 Roles of different types of lymphocyte

Cell type	Immunological role
B lymphocyte	Multiply in response to specific infections and produce antibodies (proteins called immunoglobulins) that bind to antigens on the cell surface of invading micro-organisms, thereby labelling them for destruction
T lymphocyte	Recognise, engulf and destroy body cells that have been infected, for example, by a virus; therefore tend to multiply during illness
Natural killer (NK) cell	Selectively target and destroy suspect cells, including cancerous cells

According to Cooper *et al.* (1988), stress causes or exacerbates all of Britain's top 20 fatal illnesses. High cortisol levels resulting from prolonged stress are associated with allergic responses; so allergic conditions such as eczema and asthma can be aggravated by prolonged stress. Rheumatoid arthritis, an autoimmune disorder causing painful inflammation of the joints, is also worsened by stress (Zautra 1998). Here, the effects of stress are indirect, resulting from physiological changes that occur in response to stress. In other situations, stress directly affects health, impairing our ability to fight disease. For example, bereavement (Schleifer *et al.* 1983), marital disruption (Kiecolt-Glaser and Glaser 1986) and students' examinations (Kiecolt-Glaser *et al.* 1994) all cause reduced immune functioning.

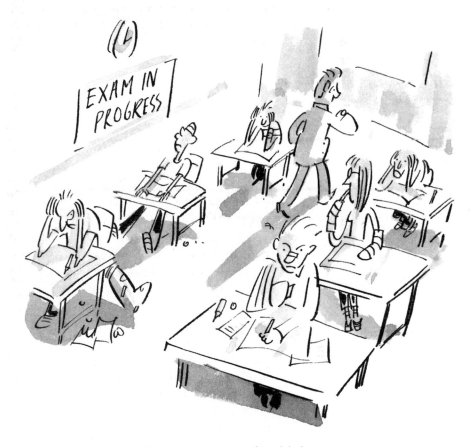

Exam stress makes students slow to recover from injuries

In addition to observing the effect of natural or experimental stressors on health, researchers can also test the effects of stress upon immune functioning when infection is induced. Cohen *et al.*

⚬—ⁿ *Keywords*
....

Saline solution
Salt water used in place of an
active solution in an
experiment

(1993) used a nasal drip to administer either a cold virus or **saline solution**. The participants were then quarantined and completed measures of their stress levels. Outcome was assessed by observing both infection (multiplication of the cold virus) and clinical disease (symptoms of a cold). Participants with high stress ratings were more likely to become infected and to develop symptoms.

In a subsequent study, Cohen *et al.* (1998) found that the risk of infection increased progressively with the duration of exposure to a stressor. A parallel effect can be demonstrated for the rate of wound healing. Students are 40% slower to recover from a standardised mechanical injury during exam time, when they are most stressed, than during vacations (Marucha *et al.* 1998).

Recent research suggests that, whilst long-term stress induces immunosuppression, resulting in an increased risk of infection and disease, short-term stress may trigger an enhancement of the immune response. In psychologically challenging situations, such as public speaking or confrontational role play, increases in natural killer cells and other lymphocytes has been observed (Evans 1998).

The explanation for these differences seems to lie in the two physiological systems controlling the stress response. The sympathetic adrenal medullary system (see page 129) seems to be temporarily activated in short-term acute stress, an effective evolutionary response enabling organisms to mobilise resources to fight possible infection caused, for example, by injury. Such elevated responses would, however, be damaging in themselves if prolonged. In contrast, one of the functions of the hypothalamic–pituitary–adrenocortical axis (see page 130), activated when stressors are chronic, is to regulate the immune system, inducing immunosuppression.

There is also considerable evidence for a link between stress and cancer although none indicates that stress *causes* cancer. Animal studies, such as that of Seligman and Visintainer (1985), have found that rates of cancer in laboratory animals increase when they are stressed. Similar results have been obtained in studies of humans. Eysenck (1988) followed up nearly 400 individuals and found that death rates from cancer were higher for those who reported greater levels of stress at the start of the study.

Normally the immune system finds and destroys cancer cells before they can establish themselves as a tumour. However, if the immune system is functioning less efficiently, then cancerous cells are less likely to be eliminated. This is arises because, as Herbert and Cohen (1993) reported, natural killer cell activity is consistently impaired by stress. Strategies such as smoking, which some people use in an attempt to reduce stress, actually make things worse by introducing **carcinogens** into the body.

⚬—ⁿ *Keywords*
....

Carcinogens
Chemicals that can cause
cancer

●━π *Keywords*

Psychoneuroimmunology
Investigates the effect of the mind on the function of the immune system and, consequently, health

Immunocompetence
The effectiveness of immune functioning

●━π *Keywords*

Metastases
Secondary cancerous growth caused by the spread of cancerous cells from an original tumour (the primary site) through the blood or lymph to other parts of the body

Psychoneuroimmunology

Psychoneuroimmunology aims to find out why an individual's attitude or state of mind affects susceptibility to, or recovery from, illness. Clearly, stress can reduce **immunocompetence**. In addition, the way an individual thinks can improve the immune response. For example, Pettingale *et al.* (1985) found that women with breast cancer who fought their illness survived, on average, 5 years longer post-diagnosis. However, Salmon (2000) observes that such personality factors may link to better survival for entirely different reasons – a person with 'fighting spirit' may eat more or may attract better care from staff because they are perkier.

Keller *et al.* (1994) suggested that the key aim for psychoneuroimmunological research was to understand the relationship between:

- Psychological distress
- Immune system functioning
- The development of disease.

In reality, few studies investigate all three of these variables simultaneously. Ben-Eliyahu *et al.* (1991) injected rats with tumour material, tested their immune function (natural killer cell level) and observed the course of the disease (the occurrence of **metastases**) under two experimental conditions (stress within 1 hour or 24 hours of the injection). They found that individuals receiving the stressor and injection together had more metastatic growth. Research such as that of Marucha *et al.* (1998), described on page 134, has succeeded in demonstrating a similar three-way relationship in humans. Immunological abnormalities have been linked to disorders such as schizophrenia, depression and Alzheimer's disease (Schwarz *et al.* 2001). The differences in such immune-related pathophysiology may lead to new, specific treatment strategies.

Life events theory

Whereas Selye's model emphasises the physiological changes associated with stress, the life events model (Holmes and Rahe 1967) attempts to link stressful events to the incidence of stress.

Holmes and Rahe initially developed a list of potentially stressful life events on which an individual could derive a score by counting the number of stressful events that had happened to them in the last year. These included minor occurrences such as 'a vacation' or 'a change in eating habits' to major traumas including 'death of a spouse' or 'personal injury or illness'. While this demonstrated links between stress and health status, it ignored differences in severity of the possible life events and was replaced by the Social Readjustment

Rating Scale (SRRS) (see Table 4.2 on page 137). Recent evidence suggests, however, that there is little difference in the power of the two scales to predict ill-health (Turner and Wheaton 1995).

Holmes and Rahe 1967

Aim: To develop a weighting system for the critical life events identified on the Scale of Recent Events.

Procedure: Records of 5000 patients were examined for life events that arose in the months preceding the onset of their illness.

Findings: Forty-three life events were found to occur often in the prescribed period. Their relative frequency was used to generate the Social Readjustment Rating Scale (SRRS). The SRRS is a list of these life events in order and weighted according to their seriousness, i.e. the relative frequency with which they were found to occur in the patients. The weightings, called life change units, can be used to calculate a score for subsequent individuals by identifying the number of significant life events that had happened to them in a specified period of time, e.g. the preceding 6 months, and adding together the value assigned to each one.

Conclusion: The SRRS can be used to predict the likelihood of a stress-related illness arising in other individuals by looking at the total of life change units. Individuals whose experiences total in excess of 300 life change units over 1 year are more likely to suffer

The SRRS includes both positive and negative events, since any deviation from the normal life pattern has the potential to be stressful. However, subsequent evidence suggested that only unpleasant events were linked to increased illness (Ross and Mirowsky 1979).

Initial evidence supported the predictive power of the SRRS. Rahe (1968) tested 2500 servicemen prior to tours of duty. The life change units were then related to medical records at the end of the first 6 months' service. Those individuals with SRRS scores in the top 30% had nearly 90% more first illnesses than those individuals in the lowest 30%.

Subsequent studies (e.g. Theorell *et al.* 1975, Goldberg and Comstock 1976), however, have not demonstrated clear relationships between stress (as indicated by the SRRS) and ill-health. This may be because ratings of life events tend to be retrospective so rely on potentially inaccuracy memories. People who are ill may perceive their lives more critically, and selectively recall negative events, or may ignore them, blaming their condition on some uncontrollable factor such as genetics, thus distorting the relationship between life events and health.

Table 4.2 The Social Readjustment Rating Scale

Rank	Life event	Mean value	Rank	Life event	Mean value
1	Death of spouse	100	23	Son or daughter leaving home	29
2	Divorce	73	24	Trouble with in-laws	29
3	Marital separation	65	25	Outstanding personal achievement	28
4	Jail term	63	26	Wife begins or stops work	26
5	Death of close family member	63	27	Begin or end school	26
6	Personal injury or illness	53	28	Change in living conditions	25
7	Marriage	50	29	Revision of personal habits	24
8	Fired at work	47	30	Trouble with boss	23
9	Marital reconciliation	45	31	Change in work hours or conditions	20
10	Retirement	45	32	Change in residence	20
11	Change in health of family member	44	33	Change in schools	20
12	Pregnancy	40	34	Change in recreation	19
13	Sex difficulties	39	35	Change in church activities	19
14	Gain of new family member	39	36	Change in social activities	18
15	Business re-adjustment	39	37	Mortgage or loan less than $10 000	17
16	Change in financial state	38			
17	Death of a close friend	37	38	Change in sleeping habits	16
18	Change to a different line of work	36	39	Change in number of family get-togethers	15
19	Change in number of arguments with spouse	35	40	Change in eating habits	15
20	Mortgage over $10 000	31	41	Vacation	13
21	Foreclosure of mortgage or loan	30	42	Christmas	12
22	Change in responsibilities at work	29	43	Minor violations of the law	11

Adding together the weightings for each event that has occurred generates a total of life change units that can be used as an indicator of the level of stress experienced.

From Holmes and Rahe 1967.

Lazarus's transactional model of stress

Lazarus suggests that an individual's experience of stress is influenced by their ability to consider the effect a stressor is having upon them. Humans can evaluate events, assessing the threat, their own vulnerability and how they might cope. From this perspective, a life event is not necessarily a source of stress; the individual's evaluation of its impact is what determines stressfulness. A student who misses a deadline but has previously been up-to-date and is confident they can catch up may be less stressed by the experience than one who knows they are about to be removed from their course for persistent tardiness. It is the perception of vulnerability and lack of control that creates a stressful situation.

Lazarus and Folkman (1984) suggest that this process of determining whether a situation is threatening, challenging or harmful is one of appraisal. Our initial impression or primary appraisal of the situation generates emotions in relation to the judgement of:

- a threat, or the anticipation of harm, generates an appraisal of fear, anxiety or worry
- harm, or damage already done, generates an appraisal of disgust, disappointment, anger or sadness
- challenge, or confidence in the face of a difficult demand, generates an appraisal of anticipation or excitement.

Following the initial appraisal, a secondary appraisal is made. This is the formation of an impression about one's ability to cope with the situation. It is a consideration of the possible options, the chances of successfully employing them and whether the action will work. A student with an overdue essay might first consider the options – copying someone else's, missing the tutorial when the work is due in, fabricating an excuse and asking for an extension, etc. They would then decide whether they could implement each action – could they lie effectively, for instance? Finally they would evaluate the chances of success – would their lecturer notice a copied essay or believe the excuse?

Reappraisal may follow in the light of new information. The student may find out that this lecturer is a pushover, or that the essay title is the same as one set last year. This knowledge would reduce the judgement of the situation from a stressful to a benign one. Alternatively, additional evidence may suggest that a previously innocent situation is a threat. The student may believe that to exceed deadlines is permissible but subsequently discover that there is a penalty for doing so.

The importance of control over the environment

A person's control over a potential stressor affects the extent of the stress response it elicits. An uncontrollable noise is, for instance, more stressful than a controllable one. This relationship can be clearly demonstrated in experimental studies with animals. Seligman and Visintainer (1985) report the effects of controllable and uncontrollable shocks on the health of rats. The experimental animals were injected with live tumour cells, then exposed to electric shocks. Tumour growth was greater in the 'uncontrollable shock' condition, suggesting that stressors that cannot be controlled by the individual and are perhaps appraised as more threatening, are more detrimental to health.

Similar results were obtained by Manuck *et al.* (1986) in their study of coronary heart disease in monkeys. Prior to the experimental manipulation, the monkeys had formed a stable hierarchy with dominant and submissive individuals. New monkeys were then introduced to destabilise the group. Since it would be harder for dominant animals to assert their position in the new social environment, they would be under greater stress; there would be a mismatch between their expectations of control and the reality of the newly developing hierarchy. The dominant animals did indeed experience a higher incidence of coronary heart disease in the unstable condition than did either dominant or submissive individuals in the stable condition.

Although animal studies may rely on assumptions of relevance to people, similar findings have emerged in relation to the human response to stressful environments. Studies in Sweden (Karasek *et al.* 1981) and in the USA (Karasek *et al.* 1988) have provided evidence suggesting that job-related stress induced by a combination of high work load, low satisfaction and little control is the best predictor of coronary heart disease. Similarly, Haynes *et al.* (1980) found that, in a group of working women, the combination of high job demand, low control and low work support was a reliable predictor of coronary heart disease. It appears that, for people as well as animals, control is vital for minimising the effects of stress on health.

Factors affecting the experience of stress

It is possible to identify particular factors that exacerbate the stress response. Biological factors may arise as a consequence of internal stressors such as pain or external ones such as the disruption of bodily rhythms. Social factors include those situations in which the source of stress is directly related to the presence of others, for instance crowded situations or arguments. Finally, psychological factors are characteristics within us, such as our personality, that affect the way in which we respond to a potentially stressful situation.

Biological factors affecting stress

Many health care professionals work shifts and this alone can be a cause of stress. Changing shifts causes a temporary **desychronisation** of the **circadian rhythm** from the local **zeitgebers** – in other words the internal body clock is working on a different cycle from external demands (such as working hours).

⊶ᴛ *Keywords*

Desynchronisation
The separation of the circadian rhythm controlled by an internal body clock from environmental stimuli such as sunrise and sunset

Circadian rhythm
A daily cycle of activity such as sleeping and waking

Zeitgeber
A regular environmental stimulus that can set the body clock

This disrupts many biological functions such as attention, gastrointestinal function and, most importantly, the sleep–wake cycle. Physiologically, these effects arise because the body clock continues to work on the previously established rhythm.

Cues such as daylight and other regular changes act as zeitgebers, setting the body clock to a new circadian rhythm. However, in the short term, shift workers must cope with the discrepancy between the body's needs and the immediate demands of their job. They will feel tired during the daytime but unable to fall asleep at night because their internal clock is out of tune.

Each time a shift is changed workers must readjust to a new schedule. For those on a night shift this is even more difficult, as the zeitgeber of daylight cannot help to synchronise their internal clock with the demands of their working hours. In addition to the biological disruption, other problems may arise if facilities and the family follow a daytime routine while the night-worker attempts to operate on a different pattern. Fenwick and Tausig (2000) found evidence for both family stress and health problems associated with working non-standard shifts.

Shift work is a characteristic of the health care profession but is detrimental to performance. Taffinder *et al.* (1998) investigated the effect of sleep deprivation on surgeons' dexterity during a simulated operation. They found that surgeons suffering overnight sleep deprivation made 20% more errors, were 14% slower than those who had had a full night's sleep and were more stressed.

Reflective activity

In their article 'A lifestyle how-to for night-shift nurses' in *Nursing Management*, Coburn and Sirois (2001) provide the following guidelines for lifestyle adjustment to help to cope with shift work:

● If possible, sleep in a dark room, with good ventilation

● To avoid discomfort, indigestion, drowsiness and weight gain, eat only small portions and avoid spicy and fatty foods when you're working nights

● Plan and communicate your social life needs – arrange breakfast dates to keep in contact

How would you justify each of the above recommendations?

Social factors affecting stress

Crowded places are generally experienced as stressful – being in a hospital waiting room, for example. Similarly, living in close proximity to others, in hospital accommodation or on a ward, is also stressful, especially for those who have not built up strategies for coping with high-density living. Many studies have investigated the stressful effects of crowding experimentally, on both humans and animals.

Calhoun (1962) studied the effect of restriction of space on rats. Under crowded conditions, dominant animals defended space and remained in better health than submissive ones. The latter became confined to a small area of the available space, were more aggressive and were abnormal in their reproductive behaviour and success (96% of offspring died before weaning). Calhoun attributed these changes to the stress of increased social interaction. Although this study does demonstrate the negative effects of crowding on social behaviour and reproduction, it does not represent natural rat behaviour, as they would not be confined in the wild but would disperse.

Christian (1955) suggested that effects of crowding such as those described above may arise as a direct consequence of stress. Christian's social stress theory proposed that high-density existence leads to social effects that are stressful, such as competition. This would result in a stress-like response mediated by the adrenal glands (pages 129–130). Disrupted hormone levels could then be directly responsible for the behavioural and physiological changes that have been identified.

To what extent are the findings from animal studies on social factors affecting stress replicated in the literature on humans? This question is difficult to answer as, although laboratory experiments into crowding are conducted, long-term investigations into the effects on humans tend to be **naturalistic observations**, meaning that the results are not directly comparable. The study described below investigates the payoff between frustrating and beneficial interactions with others, such as patients and staff may experience on wards or in hospital accommodation. Consider the implications of the findings for ward size.

⊶ฅ *Keywords*

Naturalistic observation
Systematic watching and recording of the behaviour of individuals conducting their day-to-day activities in their normal environment

Baum and Valins 1977

Aim: To investigate the balance between the benefits of increased opportunities to interact as density increases and the costs of such enforced encounters.

Procedure: The perceptions and behaviour of occupants of two different types of university hall of residence were compared. The accommodation was either corridor-style or suite-style, each offering the same amount of space per individual, number of individuals per floor and the same facilities (the bathroom and lounge). They differed only in the number of other individuals sharing those facilities (either 4–6 in suites or 34 on corridors) and hence the number of different interpersonal encounters.

continued

Findings: Residents in corridor-style accommodation perceived their floors to be more crowded. They were more likely to feel that they had to engage in inconvenient and unwanted social interactions and expressed a greater desire to avoid other people. Their feelings of helplessness were reflected in their social skills. They were less likely to initiate a conversation with a stranger, less able to reach a consensus after a discussion, less socially assertive and more likely to give up in a competitive game.

Conclusion: Exposure to a large number of other people, especially when the group lacks social structure, has negative consequences resulting in less sociable behaviour. The enforced, uncontrollable personal contacts experienced by the corridor residents were stressful and led to a feeling of helplessness so they tended to avoid social interactions and were less assertive in ambiguous situations because they had learned that they had little control over their social environment.

☛ Keywords

Social support
A coping strategy based on assistance from others, either direct helping or indirect encouragement. It can be received from people such as partners, family, friends and neighbours and from membership of organisations such as the church, as well as from pets

Crowding appears to reduce both liking for specific individuals and for social interaction in general. Furthermore, the effects of crowding on social interaction seem to reduce the ability to seek out others for help. Lepore *et al.* (1991) found that individuals who had high levels of **social support** lost this buffering effect after eight months in crowded conditions; they no longer sought the assistance of other people as a resource in times of psychological distress. Crowding results in withdrawal; it seems to erode the social support networks that are most important in stressful situations. This finding may have implications for the rehabilitation of patients after a prolonged stay in hospital.

Evans (1979) reported that varying crowding, for instance by putting 10 people in an 8-foot by 12-foot room, increased blood pressure and other physiological indicators of stress. Students living in high-density accommodation make more frequent visits to the infirmary (Baron *et al.* 1976) and Fuller *et al.* (1993) report a higher level of physical illness in crowded conditions. Thus there are implications for detrimental stress-induced effects on health not only in experimental settings but in natural ones too, suggesting that health care environments, as potential sources of stress, can add to the burden of ill-health.

Psychological factors affecting stress

Various personality factors affect the experience of stress. For example, Firth-Cozens (1997) described the role of self-criticism in health professionals. Student doctors who displayed high self-criticism were more likely to suffer from stress and depression 10 years into their careers. Firth-Cozens observes that being able to predict which individuals are most likely to suffer from stress provides the potential for intervention and prevention. Two distinct personality types have been linked to the incidence of stress. Type A personalities are more likely to suffer from the ill-effects of stress whereas people with hardy personalities are less at risk.

A further factor responsible for individual differences in responses to stress is the locus of control, the extent to which an individual attributes control to factors they can or cannot govern, i.e. whether they believe that they are responsible for what befalls them.

The type A personality

Two doctors, Friedman and Rosenman, began their research into personality with a casual observation of the state of their waiting room furniture. The pattern of wear on the chairs was unusual; rather than wearing on the seat, the front edge and arms had worn out first. They later observed that their coronary patients tended to sit on the edge of their seat, leaping up frequently to enquire how much longer they would be kept waiting for their appointments. The possibility of a connection between the heart conditions and the tense, frenetic behaviour of these individuals led to the proposal of 'hurry sickness', later re-named 'type A behaviour' (Friedman and Rosenman 1974).

It is possible to classify people into personality types on the basis of patterns of behaviour. Type A individuals tend to be highly competitive, aggressive, impatient and hostile, with a strong urge for success. Their behaviour tends to be goal directed and performed at speed. In contrast, people with type B behaviour are relatively laid back, lacking the urgency and drive typical of type A individuals. Some individuals do not fall clearly into either category and are termed type X.

The risk of stress-related illnesses, such as coronary heart disease, is greater for type A individuals than for type B (Rosenman *et al.* 1975, Haynes *et al.* 1980). Type A behaviour of itself may not necessarily cause stress; individuals with this personality type may tend to expose themselves to more stressful situations, such as high-pressure jobs, or may experience situations such as queuing as more annoying. Even if the cause is psychological, the effect must be still be mediated by a biological process. One significant difference in this respect is hostility. The tendency for people displaying type A behaviours to be aggressive may lead them to experience more conflicts with others, for example when driving. Several studies (e.g. Perry and Baldwin 2000) have found that type A behaviours are associated with aggression on the road.

Day surgery nurse

Professionally speaking . . .

Knowing what to expect – how communication helps to reduce stress

I think my job involves being able to balance physical care needs with social and psychological care. Pre-operatively I undertake the general assessment of the patients checking their general medical condition and whether they're fit for anaesthetic. I also try to determine their psychological state as well, because that will affect their recovery an awful lot. I can then advise the recovery nurse if the patient is very anxious, as this may affect their recovery and they end up in a state, thrashing about and being quite disturbed. I also find out about their social situation, and whether they've got someone at home to look after them. It's very important if you've got someone coming in for bilateral carpal tunnel surgery that they've got someone at home who can help them cope.

Communication is also vital in my job, with the surgeon and the anaesthetist, and giving the patients information.

Postoperatively I assess the patient's condition, seeing when s/he is fit for discharge and giving postoperative advice. I need to make sure s/he understands and his/her relatives understand. I make sure they've got their drugs and doctors letters and appointment letters. If necessary I may have to admit them to a ward area.

◖━┱ Keywords

Neurohormonal
Events or sequences involving interaction between the nervous and endocrine systems

Atherosclerosis
Hardening of the arteries due to fatty deposits lining the inside walls of the vessels

A possible physiological route of action is the **neurohormonal** system, specifically the effects of hormone levels on **atherosclerosis**. Type A individuals show elevated heart rate, blood pressure, skin conductance and catecholamine response. These are all changes associated with stress, resembling chronic activation of the sympathetic adrenal medullary system (see page 129).

Not all studies demonstrate a clear relationship between stress and type A behaviour. Freeman *et al.* (2000) predicted that the political violence in Northern Ireland would increase the stress experienced by members of the population and it would be expected that individuals demonstrating type A behaviours would be more severely affected. However, when Freeman *et al.* compared stress levels in groups of dental students from Belfast in 1992 and during the 1994–96 cease-fire, they found no effect related to type A behaviour. The students' personality did not seem to affect their experience of stress, although other factors, such as gender and social support, were important.

Hardiness

Kobasa (1979) studied the stress levels, personalities and health of executives. She found that, of those who were highly stressed, the individuals who did or did not become ill differed in terms of a personality factor she called hardiness. There are three key characteristics of a hardy personality. These are:

- **Commitment** –a sense of purpose and involvement in events and activities
- **Control** – a belief that one can influence event in one's own life
- **Challenge** – a perception of change as positive and representing an opportunity for growth rather than a threat.

The hardy executives were less ill, perhaps because they treated problems as potentially beneficial and therefore less stressful. As a result they may take more direct action in the face of stress, such as problem-focused coping strategies (see page 153), enabling them to tackle rather than avoid issues. Recent evidence suggests that a hardy personality may also reduce the likelihood of 'burnout' when under pressure (Sciacchitano *et al.* 2001).

Korbasa's original study only looked at males, although subsequent investigations have demonstrated similar effects in women. Rhodewalt and Zone (1989) assessed the illness and depression ratings of women with high and low hardiness scores. They found that hardy women suffered lower rates of illness and depression following undesirable life changes than non-hardy women. The women also differed in their interpretation of life changes. High and low hardiness scorers experienced similar numbers of stressful events but more were classified as undesirable by the non-hardy group. This suggests that hardy individuals appraise potentially stressful events differently, buffering them against the negative effects of stress.

Hardiness may, however, be explained without recourse to special features of hardy people. First, it may be nothing more than positive **affect**. The effects of better coping might simply be explained by more positive appraisal and interpretation of events in the individual's life. Alternatively, hardiness may have an indirect rather than a direct effect on illness. 'Hardy' individuals may be more likely to engage in successful health-related behaviours, thus having a lower risk of illness.

Locus of control

There is good evidence that having control over one's situation is a contributory factor in illness and health, for example in relation to the hypothalamic–pituitary–adrenocortical axis (page 130) and lack of control in crowded environments (page 141). Langer and Rodin (1976) showed that the simple manipulation of personal control in elderly clients in a retirement home affected their health and longevity. Langer and Rodin manipulated control by giving the

o—π *Keywords*

Affect
In the context of psychology this refers to emotions or feelings

clients a talk, a plant for their room and the opportunity to see a film. In the experimental group the talk stressed personal responsibility, the individuals were asked where they would like the plant put and which night they would like to see the film. The other groups' talk did not focus on responsibility and they were told – rather than asked – where the plant would be placed and when they would see the film. The residents who experienced greater control were happier and healthier and more active, alert and sociable and, 18 months later, their death rate was only 15% compared with 30% for the comparison group. These findings suggest that control, or the perception of control, may be an important factor in determining health with implications for the importance of enabling patients to have control over aspects of their own environment and care.

Reflective activity

Reflect on the choices you have made about the environment in which you live and sleep, the food you eat, when you sleep and wake up, and the company you keep. Now consider how many of those factors are determined for patients by hospital regimes. Can you think of examples of ways in which patients are, or could be, given control?

The way individuals appraise their role in controlling their own lives also appears to be important. Rotter (1966) identified a personality variable he called the locus of control. People who attribute control to factors they cannot govern, such as chance or the behaviour of other people, are described as having an external locus of control. Those who believe that they are responsible for themselves have an internal locus of control. This internal–external dimension may also relate to health behaviour. Strickland (1978) suggested that individuals with an internal locus of control may engage in more preventative measures such as avoiding accidents and being informed about their own health.

The precise role of locus of control in the context of health has been investigated using the health locus of control (HLC) scale developed by Wallston *et al.* (1978). This measure, which looks specifically at an individual's beliefs about the factors that determine their health outcomes, assesses three dimensions:

- **Internal health locus of control** – the extent to which the individual feels able to be responsible for their own health, for instance believing that 'the main thing that affects my health is what I myself do'

- **Powerful others' control over health** – the individual's belief in the role that other, important, people (such as doctors, nurses, family and friends) play in their health and holds views such as 'Whenever I don't feel well, I should consult a trained professional'
- **Chance health locus of control** – the role that the individual assigns to pure 'luck' (or otherwise) and indicated by beliefs such as 'No matter what I do, if I am going to get sick, I will get sick'.

Norman *et al.* (1998) investigated the link between HLC and health-related behaviour. They surveyed 11 000 people using the three factors listed above and recorded the individuals' health behaviours, including smoking, alcohol use, exercise and diet. Participants with an internal HLC engaged in more health-protective behaviours but those with mixtures of high and low scores on the three measures were less health-conscious, suggesting that effective health promotion may need to use a range of strategies to target individuals with differing beliefs about the determinants of their health.

Steptoe and Wardle 2001

Aim: To investigate the relationship between health locus of control (HLC), health values and health-related behaviours in a diverse sample.

Procedure: A total of 4358 female and 2757 male university students aged 18–30 years from 18 European countries were tested on three measures: HLC, health values and 10 health-related behaviours (physical exercise, not smoking, limited alcohol consumption, regular breakfast, daily tooth-brushing, seat-belt use and consumption of fruit, fat, fibre and salt).

Findings: There was a significant difference in the behaviours exhibited by individuals with the highest compared to the lowest internal HLC scores. Those with the lowest scores were 40% more likely to engage in five of the health-compromising behaviours (exercise, daily tooth-brushing, eating fibre and avoiding salt and fat). Similarly, those with the highest chance HLC scores were 20% less likely to select the healthy option for more than half of the behaviours (not smoking, limited alcohol consumption, regular breakfast, daily fruit, eating fibre and avoiding fat).

Conclusion: Low internal HLC and high chance HLC are associated with poor health choices. A low internal score suggests that the individual does not believe that they can affect their own health for the better, so they do not try. A high chance score indicates that the individual believes that factors outside their control influence their health and that their own efforts are therefore irrelevant.

Support for the HLC was also obtained by O'Carroll *et al.* (2001) in relation to the response of individuals who had suffered a myocardial infarction (heart attack). Many patients fail to request help when they are having a heart attack and O'Carroll *et al.* found that a high chance HLC was the best predictor of delay in seeking medical attention. Because these individuals believe that chance is a major factor determining their health (rather than, say, their own actions) they do not seek help soon enough and their delay, in these circumstances, could be fatal. O'Carroll *et al.* suggest that attempts to modify the beliefs of people at risk could reduce their response time and therefore increase survival rates.

Many people engage in health-compromising behaviours such as drug-taking, unprotected sex or overeating. Individuals with a high score on the chance dimension of HLC, whose beliefs suggest that whatever they do will have little effect on their health, would be expected to be less aware of, or ignore, risks to health. Hodgson (2001) used a student population to investigate perceived risk, risk-taking behaviour and HLC. The results showed a link between these variables, suggesting that – for adolescents at least – those who believe that their health status is determined by chance factors are more likely to engage in risky activities. This identifies a high risk group in terms of their age, occupation and beliefs and provides the basis for specifically targeted health education.

Key points | Top tips

Stress is increased by a range of biological, social and psychological factors:

- Shift work disrupts bodily rhythms, affecting sleep and concentration
- Crowding can make people more aggressive, less helpful and withdrawn, so they are less likely to seek help
- Personality can influence susceptibility to the negative effects of stress; type A people and those who are less hardy are more likely to become ill when stressed
- Locus of control is a measure of beliefs about the source of the reasons for and solutions to ill health. Individuals with an internal locus of control may be advantaged in dealing with the effects of stress.

Consequences of stress

Effects of stressors on health

Clearly, stress has a detrimental effect on health via its impact on the endocrine and immune systems. In addition, some stressors have direct effects on health, such as damage from loud noise (above 150 dB), which can rupture the eardrum, but permanent hearing loss can also arise through damage to the sensitive hair cells of the inner ear (which detect sound) at 90–120 dB, such as experienced in loud working environments. Cohen *et al.* (1973) found that children in a high-rise block living closest to the traffic below had significantly impaired hearing. In addition to the obvious effects of noise, it can also cause raised blood pressure and other effects associated with stress.

Another environmental stressor, pollution, has direct biological effects on health – lead can cause brain and liver damage, arsenic is a carcinogen, ozone aggravates respiratory problems, etc. In addition, pollution can have indirect psychological effects on wellbeing. Air pollution may prevent us from going out, and may increase the risk of aggression and reduce the likelihood of helping behaviour (Jones and Bogat 1978, Cunningham 1979). Furthermore, the stressful effects of major life events seem to be exacerbated by air pollution (Evans *et al.* 1987).

Cardiovascular disorders

The effects of chronic stress include **hypertension** and atherosclerosis (build up of fat deposits in blood vessels). Hypertension is a direct result of high levels of aldosterone and high levels of fat in the blood caused by elevated cortisol levels contribute to atherosclerosis. Both atherosclerosis and hypertension can cause serious problems in themselves but they also increase the probability of having a heart attack or stroke. Talbott *et al.* (1990) compared men working in relatively noisy and quiet employment and reported a positive correlation between hearing loss and raised blood pressure. Comparing men from each setting who had worked there for 15 years, blood pressure was in general higher for those in noisier settings. This shows that workers exposed to the stressor of noise for a prolonged period of time suffer an increased risk of cardiovascular disorders.

In simulated situations Maschke *et al.* (1995) have demonstrated that noisy work environments increase the level of adrenaline. Evans *et al.* (1995) found similar results with children; those living close to a noisy airport had higher levels of adrenaline (epinephrine) and noradrenaline (norepinephrine) and higher blood pressure compared to those living further away. The use of protective equipment at work can, however, reduce noise perception, lowering both adrenaline levels and blood pressure (Ising and Melchert 1980). Job dissatisfaction exacerbates the effects of noise at work. Lercher *et al.* (1993) found that annoyance was related to both noise levels in the workplace and blood pressure and that this link was stronger in dissatisfied workers.

Gastrointestinal disorders

Stress is associated with a number of gastrointestinal disorders. The sensation of 'butterflies in the stomach' is not dangerous in itself but, if we experience it regularly, it is likely to interfere with our eating patterns. Stress also causes high levels of hydrochloric acid in the stomach. This is believed to contribute to the development of stomach and duodenal ulcers. However, while there is still a popular belief among doctors and the general public that stress causes ulcers (Novelli 1997), there is now good evidence that stress is not the major cause of stomach ulcers – they are the result of bacterial infection (Macarthur *et al.* 1995). Harris (1999) suggests that the symptoms of irritable bowel syndrome (which includes constipation and diarrhoea) are worsened by episodes of stress.

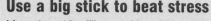

media watch   Use a big stick to beat stress

More than 13 million working days were lost last year because of stress, which affects one in five employees, at a cost of £3.8 billion, according to the Health and Safety Executive (HSE). A recent survey by the insurance company Union Provident revealed that stress-related illnesses have overtaken back pain as Britain's most common workplace ailment.

The HSE has just taken the ground-breaking step of ordering an NHS trust to improve its methods of tackling stress, after an inspector visited Dorset County Hospital in Dorchester, following a complaint from a member of staff. Although, for reasons of confidentiality, no details of the complaint were released, failure to comply with the order could result in the trust being prosecuted and fined. Next year, a tough code will be introduced by the HSE which will see all employers at risk of legal action if they ignore the issue of stress.

'Quite apart from minor ailments, such as headaches and back pain, ultimately, stress can lead to a heart attack or mental illness, and there's a lot of research going on into whether it is related to cancer,' says Howard Kahn, a senior lecturer on organisational psychology at Heriot–Watt University in Edinburgh.

'An individual can go swimming, take up yoga or give up smoking, but if he or she still has to go to the same lousy, stressful job morning after morning, it won't make that much difference,' he says.

Typical symptoms of stress include constant tiredness, lack of energy and aching limbs. Headaches, colds, stomach problems, and back and neck pain are also common.

Public workers such as nurses and teachers typically suffer from the highest rates of stress, depression and anxiety, as the private sector is often more proactive in seeking to alleviate stress. But although these inventive measures to combat the effects of stress sound admirable, they beg the question: Why not stop staff becoming stressed in the first place?

Of course, it would be simplistic to suggest that a couple of hours' drumming or a few Pilates sessions is all it would take to restore morale to overworked NHS nurses or boost teachers bogged down by bureaucracy. Nevertheless, stress-relief activities do have a useful role in some office environments, where staff are encouraged to take regular breaks to avoid burnout.

Edited from an article by Judith Woods, *Daily Telegraph*, 10 September 2003; accessed online at: www.telegraph.co.uk

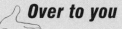

> ### Over to you
>
> What evidence could you present to support the negative effects of stress on health suggested in the article?

Effects of stressors on performance

Performance at work is affected by environmental stressors such as noise, not just in obviously loud settings such as construction sites and airports but in other workplaces too. Banbury and Berry (1998) suggest that the background noise generated by voices, such as is experienced on a busy ward, is particularly troublesome. Because we tend to 'tune-in' to conversations, they are more likely to interfere with our own concentration and communication. Acton (1970) found that we can, however, learn to adapt to working in a noisy environment. Workers from an industrial setting, accustomed to higher noise levels, were more effective at communicating against a background of loud noise than were university employees, whose workplaces are typically quieter.

Effects of stressors on social behaviour

As noise can affect attention, arousal and stress, it is likely to have an effect on social interactions. It seems to make people unpleasant; they are more aggressive and less helpful. Sauser *et al.* (1978) found that participants exposed to a loud noise during a management simulation were likely to assign lower salaries to fictitious job applicants. Loud noise also seems to reduce the probability of altruistic behaviour. Page (1977) conducted a field experiment in which a pedestrian (a **confederate**) dropped a package near a construction site. Under different noise conditions created with a pneumatic drill, the incidence of passers-by stopping to help was recorded. Fewer passers-by helped in noisy conditions, especially when it was very loud.

Mathews and Canon (1975) investigated the interaction between the effect of noise on helping behaviour and another factor known to influence the likelihood of altruism, apparent need. The experimenters contrived a situation in which a pedestrian dropped some books on a city street. Two variables were manipulated in the staged incidents; whether the pedestrian's arm was in a cast, and noise generated by a nearby lawn-mower. Although the noise reduced altruism in both conditions, the effect was most marked in the reduction of offers of help when the pedestrian's arm was in a cast.

⊙━ₐ Keywords

Confederate

An individual in an experiment who appears to be a participant but is actually an assistant to the researcher

Such results arise because people attend to fewer social cues under conditions of sensory overload – participants in Matthews and Canon's 'noisy' condition may not have noticed the cast. Alternatively, the noise may affect mood, making people less inclined to help when in a noisy environment.

From the results of a study conducted by Yinon and Bizman (1980), mood seems to be less important than attention. Participants' mood was manipulated by giving them positive or negative feedback on a task they had performed. During the task, they were exposed to either loud or quiet noise. Finally, the participants were asked for help (by a confederate). If noise affected altruism by having a detrimental effect on mood, it would be expected that the combination of loud noise and a negative report on performance would reduce the likelihood of helping. However, Yinon and Bizman found that in the loud noise condition there was no difference between helping by participants who had received positive or negative feedback. As there was a difference in the low noise condition these results suggest that the effect of the loud noise over-rides that of feedback, either distracting the participants from the negative feedback or justifying it. It seems that interference from a stressor such as noise is more important than mood in determining social behaviour. So, for health carers in a busy, noisy department, the environment may detract from their ability to assist patients effectively.

The environmental stressor of air pollution, in particular cigarette smoke, can affect social behaviour. In a study of office productivity, Harris *et al.* (1980) found that 35% of workers smoked and that the smoking of nearby co-workers distressed 26% of the non-smoking majority. In a shopping centre, people on public benches left more quickly if a smoker, rather than a non-smoker, joined them (Bleda and Bleda 1978). Jones and Bogat (1978) found that volunteers would administer higher levels of aversive noise to another person if they were exposed to cigarette smoke. These responses could be due to a direct physiological response to chemicals in the smoke itself or to the annoyance it causes. Nonetheless, such findings support hospitals' insistence on 'no smoking' policies.

Coping with stress

Coping represents the ways in which we attempt to deal with aspects of the world that we find are beyond our normal means to fight. One way in which people attempt to cope with stress is through the unconscious use of defence mechanisms, as proposed

⊶ꞮꞮ Keywords

Coping
An individual's cognitive and behavioural attempts to manage (limit, overcome or tolerate) internal and external demands in the physical and social environment that are judged to be challenging or beyond that individual's resources

by Sigmund Freud (1894). The individual protects themselves from painful, frightening or guilty feelings that could cause stress, by unconsciously denying access to those thoughts or changing the way that they are interpreted. These mechanisms include:

- **Displacement** – the redirecting of emotions
- **Regression** – the use of childlike strategies to comfort ourselves
- **Repression** – the blocking of a memory so that it cannot be recalled.

If a stressful situation, such as an argument at home, makes an individual angry, they may use displacement and express their anger on other people, such as colleagues. Alternatively, they may become difficult – acting like a child – and use regression to avoid having to deal with the real issues. It is not uncommon in severe cases of stress, such as a traumatised road accident patient, to have no recollection of the stressful events themselves; this would be described as repression.

Stress management strategies

Sources of stress can be tackled from an external or internal perspective, that is, coping strategies can be either problem focused, aiming to reduce the causes of stress; or emotion focused, aiming to manage the negative effects on the individual. In any situation, a combination of these strategies may be employed.

Problem–focused strategies

Problem-focused strategies include discussing the situation with a professional, relying on one's own past experiences to tackle the issue and dealing with the situation one step at time.

Emotion–focused strategies

Emotion-focused strategies include keeping busy to take one's mind off the problem, preparing oneself for the worst, praying for strength and guidance, ignoring the situation in the belief that the problem will go away and bottling feelings up. Other strategies are listed in Table 4.3.

How effective are the strategies?

It seems obvious that problem-focused strategies are better because they deal with the cause. However, it may be beyond the scope of the individual to effect change, so emotion-focused solutions may be essential to enable the individual to feel less stressed about the situation. For example, a patient could not reverse an accidental amputation, nor could a bereaved relative bring back their loved one.

Table 4.3 Some examples of strategies that may be employed in response to environmental stressors (N.B. These are not intended to represent the best ways to cope!)

Source of stress	Emotion-focused strategy	Problem-focused strategy
Noisy children playing in the waiting area	Trying to remember that children need to play and it's good for them to be active (being objective)	Talking to a friend on the telephone about it in the evening (discussing the situation)
Smoke coming in the window from a bus stop below	Snapping at patients (taking anger out on others)	Closing the window (taking positive action)
You're on a night shift trying to work with the lights down but you can't concentrate because your desk lamp keeps flickering so you have to stop	Accepting that you'd probably make a better job of it tomorrow anyway (seeing positive side of situation)	Taking the opportunity to request a new bulb as well as gloves and bags that were also running out (considering alternative solutions)
You arrive on shift and the laundry room is a total mess	Eating or smoking more (trying to reduce tension)	Trying to find out who was responsible on the previous shift (investigating the issue)

Cultural factors also affect coping. Frydenberg *et al.* (2003) compared the way in which young people from different cultures dealt with their concerns. They found that, although all adolescents seemed to cope by working hard – perhaps to 'take their mind off the problem' – there were some differences. For example, Palestinian students focused more on social support, spiritual support and worrying than Australian and German students, who rated physical recreation highly among their coping strategies. Such differences suggest that it may be important to ensure that coping strategies made available to patients reflect cultural values.

Reflective activity

Identify examples from your placement of patients (or staff) using emotion-focused and problem-focused coping strategies

In some situations emotion-focused strategies are detrimental; evidence suggests that long-term avoidance may be ineffective (Nolen-Hoeksema and Larson 1999). Avoidance strategies may even be damaging. Epping-Jordan *et al.* (1994) found that, in patients using avoidance strategies, the progression of cancer was faster.

> ### Over to you
>
> There are occasions when, although taking action to reduce stress would be ideal, it is simply not possible – for example if you are a patient awaiting a diagnosis or a health care worker whose patience is frayed. What can be done to regain control? Rationalising the situation can help. Imagine a situation in which you are due for an annual review meeting with your manager but there has been a crisis on the ward and you know you will miss the appointment. What cognitive strategies would you use?
>
> - **Informational control** – find out as much as you can about the situation – how annoyed will your manager be? Will it affect the outcome of your appraisal?
>
> - **Decisional control** – make a choice and stick to it – get on with it, pray, or try to get a message to your appraiser
>
> - **Cognitive control** – rationalise the situation – perhaps you could arrange to have the meeting rescheduled? – or recognise that, even if you had gone, you would have done badly as your mind would have been elsewhere
>
> - **Retrospective control** – reflect on the way you reacted, decide what you have gained – maybe that you should book important events outside your working hours or that you value patients more than meetings.

Resources to help with stress management

Different individuals, circumstances or situations may lead to the availability of differing resources to assist with coping. Wealth may offer the means to overcome many stressors (through avoidance or protection) but it may not provide a solution to inescapable sources of stress. Here, intrapersonal resources may be of greater significance. Wealth has been demonstrated to be linked to reduced stress but this does not apply to everyone (tending only to be important at the lower end of the socioeconomic scale, Dohrenwend 1973). Neither is wealth a buffer against all sources of stress; it is not particularly important following bereavement, for example (Stroebe and Stroebe 1987).

Social resources

People gain help, reassurance and assistance from their interactions with others (including their pets), which helps them to deal with stress; this is called social support. As we saw on page 144, one way that people help to combat the stress of living in a time of political violence is to rely on support from others. How can an individual's social contacts provide support during stressful experiences? The kinds of support offered by social networks has been categorised in a

Table 4.4 Resources for coping with stressors

Type of resource	Examples	Ways they might be employed
Material	Wealth	Having more money might enable people to pay for private health insurance and avoid stressful delays
Educational	Published research (including posters, leaflets and media information) schools, Internet	Knowing how to find recipes for meals with low salt or fat content
Physical	Strength, health	Individuals without asthma may be more tolerant of some air pollutants
Intrapersonal	Skills, abilities and personality characteristics such as determination and self-esteem	One individual might be better able to work effectively on a crowded ward than another
Social	Family, friends, pets, neighbours, community organisations	Being able to talk to the family dog about an impending operation may alleviate some of the fears about the procedure

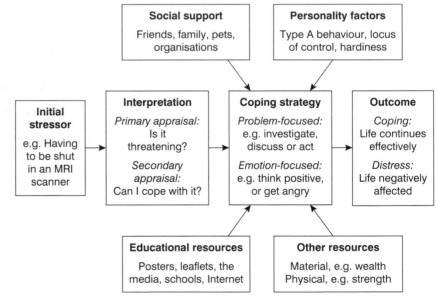

Coping with stress

number of different ways (e.g. Cohen and Wills 1985, Stroebe and Stroebe 1987). These are summarised by Stroebe (2000):

- **Emotional support** – providing empathy, care, love and trust
- **Instrumental support** – direct help such as caring for children or offering transport

- **Informational support** – providing routes to knowledge and understanding that will help individuals to cope with their problems
- **Appraisal support** – providing information that will specifically help the individual's self-evaluation, such as being able to compare oneself to another individual.

Over to you

Consider the following potential social resources that could relieve stress for someone enduring a personal crisis such as a diagnosis of a terminal disease. How would you categorise them using the Stroebe (2000) model?

Money, companionship, encouragement, leaflets about the problem, doing their washing, finding case studies of other people with similar difficulties, giving them web addresses for Internet support groups, offering compliments that boost their self-esteem, taking them to local groups dealing with their issues.

One source of social support for health professionals is the other members of their team. Carter and West (1999) found that NHS employees who worked within a clearly defined team were less likely to suffer from stress, and they also reported greater job satisfaction and commitment than among those who did not work in a team. They suggest that team work helps people to cope by providing clear goals, an understanding of expectations and higher social support. Importantly, team members can provide a buffer against the negative effects of the working environment, such as poor communication and co-operation and a lack of resources and training.

Social support can be measured in two ways:

- Perceived support considers the respondent's description of individuals they could rely upon for assistance, such as who they could discuss an intimate problem with or ask for advice
- Received support is the actual frequency with which an individual has gained specific supportive behaviours from others.

These two measures appear to be linked, but the relationship is not strong (e.g. Dunkel-Schetter and Bennett 1990). This may be the consequence of the ways in which different individuals use others to assist them – talking to one person often or many people occasionally, for example. Surprisingly, perceived support may be a better predictor of health status than actual support.

Studying actual support is relatively simple; the inventory of socially supportive behaviours (Barrera *et al.* 1981) asks respondents about specific supportive behaviours in the domains of emotional, tangible, cognitive-informational and direct guidance support. An average is generated for each respondent based on the total number of occurrences of such assistance in the previous 4 weeks. Perceived support can also be assessed using questionnaires, such as the interpersonal support evaluation list (ISEL; Cohen *et al.* 1985). The ISEL measures four sources of social support: tangible, appraisal, self-esteem and belonging.

There is good evidence to show that social support is an important variable in health status. For example, Berkman and Syme (1979) found that those individuals with low social support had roughly twice the mortality risk of high scoring individuals over the 9 years following assessment of their initial health and social support.

Professionally speaking . . .

What stress-related issues do you commonly encounter?

Occupational health nurse

Generally the symptoms displayed by health workers who are stressed are more emotional and behavioural, rather than physical, although we have many health care workers with back problems that are often linked to stress.

To be able to initiate a problem-focused strategy the health care worker's 'emotional' state needs to be addressed, either with counselling, changing mind set, etc. then moving on to a problem-focused strategy can be useful.

Time management and prioritising workload is always beneficial to staff. It also helps if they belong to a supportive team and have access to a helpful mentor.

Berkman and Syme used subjective self-report measures of health status. However, in a subsequent study, House *et al.* (1982) used more objective measures of health. These included testing blood pressure, cholesterol level and respiratory function, and electrocardiography. They, too, found that after a 10–12-year follow-up period, the mortality risk was approximately double for people with a low level of social support.

One explanation of how social support affects health is the buffering hypothesis. This proposes that social support protects the individual from the negative effects of stress, either by enabling socially supported individuals to appraise stressful situations differently or by enhancing their ability to cope with the stressor. For example, an effective social network may enable stressed individuals to appraise a physical disability in a less damaging way because they recognise that they have people who can offer them advice or financial assistance. Alternatively, individuals may deal with the disability better precisely because they have those sources of advice and assistance.

If the buffering hypothesis is correct, the effects of social support should only be seen when stress levels are high. This is rather like the consequence of inoculation against a disease; if you have an influenza injection you appear identical to someone who has not, until you are exposed to the 'flu virus – under these conditions, your vaccination protects you against the disease. Likewise, buffering would only come into effect when the stressed individual's own resources were insufficient. DeLongis *et al.* (1988) investigated the stress levels, self-esteem and health of 75 married couples. Those individuals in unsupportive relationships (i.e. low social support) with low self-esteem became more ill in stressful situations than did individuals in supportive relationships with high self-esteem.

An alternative to the buffering hypothesis, the main effect hypothesis, suggests that an absence of social support is in itself stressful and is the cause (rather than the consequence) of ill health. Social encounters are often positive and rewarding experiences and community membership can provide us with a sense of belonging and raise our self-esteem. This would imply that social support would be important to health regardless of stress levels. Hence the main effect hypothesis would predict that people with stronger social networks should be healthier regardless of the stressors they encounter.

The main effect hypothesis is also supported by empirical evidence. Lin *et al.* (1979) investigated the relationship between social support and psychiatric symptoms. They used information about participants' interactions with friends and neighbours and their community involvement as measures of social support. They found that those individuals with higher levels of social contact had lower levels of psychiatric symptoms irrespective of their stress levels. This supports the main effect hypothesis. However, as this was a **correlational** study, it is possible that individuals with psychiatric symptoms found it more difficult to establish or maintain social contacts; causality between the two variables cannot be determined.

It would appear that, when social support is measured as the absolute number of different social contacts that could be relied upon, results appear to be consistent with the main effect hypothesis. However, if social support is assessed functionally, in

o—ᴎ *Keywords*
....

Correlation
A relationship between two variables in which a change in one variable is associated with (but cannot be said to cause) a change in the other

terms of the roles that social contacts can play in offering support, the buffering hypothesis is supported (Bishop 1994).

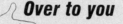

Over to you

Social support may help people to cope with a critical experience such as being an injured survivor of a traumatic event like a rail crash. Consider the two explanations for the beneficial effect of social support and decide which would suggest that people with high social support would benefit more in this situation than when exposed to day-to-day hassles.

Educational resources

One way that the effects of stress on health can be mediated is through information, as knowledge underlies our health beliefs and attitudes, so is important (although not exclusively so) to the development of health behaviours. One of the roles of educational resources is therefore to provide knowledge and understanding about the health behaviour of individuals under stress and to suggest strategies they may employ to minimise and cope with stressors and reduce the associated health risks. Chapter 2 describes theories that explain how our health behaviours are controlled and discusses health education in detail.

Over to you

If you have already studied the concepts in Chapter 2, you might like to use them to consider how you would plan a strategy for helping to reduce stress – *before* reading on.

The Mental Health Foundation, the Health Education Board for Scotland and the Royal College of Psychiatrists, among many others, provide educational information about stress. Broadly, this information covers:

- Explaining what stress is
- The effects or symptoms of stress
- Why being stressed is a problem
- The causes of stress
- Potential ways to deal with stress.

Educating people to the risks of stress enables them to make informed decisions about combating the effects of stress on their health. In order to do this they must be aware both of the causes of stress that they are experiencing and the possible courses of action they can take to reduce the stressors or minimise their effects. Thus information about sources of stress and positive courses of action are very important especially to the deployment of problem-focused strategies (see page 153). In addition, such information would provide the basis for judgements of perceived vulnerability to stress and seriousness of its effects, perceived barriers to taking action against stress and benefits of doing so. These components form the basis of health belief model (see page 58).

Explaining about stress

One factor that affects an individual's ability to cope with stress is his or her understanding of the condition or situation. Educational information about stress can help people to feel that they can overcome their condition as it offers a means to gain control. According to both the theory of planned behaviour (pages 64–68) and self-empowerment approaches (see page 79) an individual's perceived behavioural control or self-efficacy is important in following through health behaviours. The role of control is also important in understanding why some individuals become more stressed than others, for instance in locus of control theory (see page 145).

media watch

What is stress?

Stress can be defined as the way you feel when you're under abnormal pressure. For example, if you are speaking in public for the first time, if you are rushing to catch the last train home, or if you are made redundant.

All sorts of situations can cause stress. The most common, however, involve work, money matters and relationships with partners, children or other family members. Stress may be caused either by major upheavals and life events such as divorce, unemployment, moving house and bereavement, or by a series of minor irritations such as feeling undervalued at work or dealing with difficult children. Sometimes there are no obvious causes.

Stressful events that are outside the range of normal human experience, for example, being abused or tortured, may lead to post-traumatic stress disorder (PTSD). . . .

Some stress can be positive and research has suggested that a moderate level of stress makes us perform better. It also makes us more alert and can help us in challenging situations such as job interviews or public speaking. Stressful situations can also be exhilarating and some people actually thrive on the excitement that comes with dangerous sports or other 'high-risk' activities.

But stress is only healthy as a short-lived response. Excessive or prolonged stress can lead to illness and physical and emotional exhaustion. Taken to extremes, stress can be a killer.

From the Mental Health Foundation website (www.mentalhealth.org.uk)

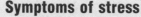

> ### Over to you
>
> Which psychological theories explain the descriptions of stress given in the extract above?

Symptoms of stress

Informing people about the effects or symptoms of stress has two benefits. Those people who are aware that they are suffering from stress may be reassured that the symptoms they are experiencing are 'normal' (i.e. characteristic of stress) and shared by others. In addition, individuals who are suffering from stress but are unaware of their condition would benefit from information to identify the problem. They may have feared that their symptoms were due to some other condition about which they may have worried unduly. In both cases information may allow the individual to take action to protect themselves from stressors in order to avoid their symptoms. According to the health belief model, knowledge about symptoms that an individual was already suffering with would indicate to them the extent of their vulnerability and hence might encourage them to take steps to protect themselves.

media watch

Symptoms of stress

Stress can damage physical health, social relationships and the way we function at work and at home. It is important to remember that the following symptoms may have nothing to do with stress but they are often danger signals which should not be ignored:

- Physical signs like headaches, insomnia, indigestion, high blood pressure
- Behaviour aspects such as poor work performance, accidents, poor relationships at home and work, dependence on tobacco, drugs and alcohol
- Emotional factors such as irritability, lack of concentration, anxiety, depression.

Mental and physical ill health are a personal loss to your employees and a cost to your company whether they mean sick pay for those who stay home or poor performance from those who come to work. A quick response can prevent the situation deteriorating further and may well lead to considerable improvements for both you and your employees.

From the Health Education Board for Scotland website (www.hebs.scot.nhs.uk)

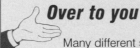

> ### Over to you
>
> Many different symptoms of stress are described above; how can they be accounted for?
>
> How might a stressed person recognise their vulnerability to stress after reading this information?

Why stress matters

Modern society is competitive and success is valued highly compared to, say, community-driven ideals. As a consequence, we may believe that stress is an inevitable part of people's lives so may be reluctant to act in response to rising stressors. This inertia can result in chronic stress responses that can be very harmful (see page 133). Educating people about the risks of stress enables them to take action against the effects of the stressors on their health, so educational strategies aiming to tackle stress need to challenge the role played by society in passively accepting stress as a consequence of modern life.

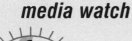

media watch

Why stress matters

Mental ill-health or distress is a major cause of sickness absence from work, reduced productivity and staff turnover. Stress is the root cause of a lot [of] mental ill-health, especially anxiety and depression.

- Work-related stress is estimated to be the biggest occupational health problem in the UK, after musculoskeletal disorders such as back problems
- Nearly three in every 10 employees will have a mental health problem in any one year – the great majority of which will be anxiety and depressive disorders
- Mental health problems account for the loss of over 91 million working days each year
- Half of all days lost through mental ill-health are due to anxiety and stress conditions.

Stress is a necessary part of everyday life. Indeed, some degree of stress or pressure is considered healthy. Underemployment can lead to boredom, apathy and a loss of energy and motivation. But conversely, excessive stress lead[s] to fatigue, impaired judgement and decision making, exhaustion and the onset of serious health problems – both mental and physical.

Physically, stress is implicated in the development of coronary heart disease, certain types of cancer, and a host of other ailments including stomach ulcers, skin rashes, migraine, asthma, and increased susceptibility to infections.

The psychological effects of stress can be just as damaging. Increased anxiety, irritability, disturbed sleep, poor concentration and aggressive behaviour can increase the risk of accidents and disrupt relationships both at work and at home. Individuals under stress are often inclined to smoke more, drink more alcohol and consume excessive amounts of caffeine, thus increasing irritability, sleep impairment, etc. in a vicious circle. Exposure to prolonged stress will increase the risk of serious mental health problems, including depression and disabling anxiety conditions, as well as alcohol misuse.

From *Mental Health in the Workplace*, a booklet from the Mental Health Foundation. Accessed online at www.mentalhealth.org.uk

Causes of stress

In order for people to improve their health behaviours they need to be aware of the causes of stress that they are experiencing. This will enable them to avoid or reduce these stressors so preventing themselves from becoming chronically stressed. Again, the health belief model would suggest that such advice should, in order to be most effective, indicate the benefits to the individual in changing their health behaviours.

media watch

What can give rise to stress at work?

- Lack of control over work
- Underutilisation of skills
- Too high a workload, no or few challenges
- Low task variety
- High uncertainty, e.g. due to poorly defined roles and responsibilities, lack of clear priorities and targets, job insecurity
- Low pay
- Poor working conditions, e.g. noise, overcrowding, excessive heat, inadequate breaks
- Low interpersonal support, e.g. via inadequate or insensitive management, hostility from colleagues
- Undervalued social position.

From *Mental Health in the Workplace*, a booklet from the Mental Health Foundation. Accessed online at www.mentalhealth.org.uk

Potential ways to deal with stress

When people have sufficient understanding of their own stress and its causes they need to know how to take appropriate action. The final role of education about stress is to inform people about the possible courses of action they can take to reduce the stressors or minimise their effects. In order for individuals to benefit from such resources, once they know that they are available, they must feel able to access them. Stress education must aim to break down the barriers that exist to seeking help in these circumstances. This is important as, according to the health belief model, people will fail to change their health behaviours if the barriers they perceive are greater than the perceived benefits.

media watch

Coping with stress

There are several things that you can do to help yourself cope. For things that happen every day, it can be useful to think of your stress as a puzzle to be solved:

- Think about the situations that stress you, and how you behave.
- Think about how you could behave differently in these situations, so that you would feel more in control of them.
- Imagine how other people might behave if you acted differently.
- List all the things you can think of that would make things easier or less stressful – write them down on a piece of paper. This can help you sort things out in your head.

Where can I get help?

Sometimes stress gets on top of you. Especially when the situation causing the stress goes on and on, and the problems just seem to keep building up. You can feel quite trapped, as if there is no way out and no solution to your problems. If you feel like this, it is important to get help.

People you might want to talk to:

- parents, a family member or family friend
- a close friend or carer
- a school nurse, teacher or school counsellor
- a social worker or youth counsellor

Your general practitioner or practice nurse may also be able to help. They may suggest that you see someone from your local child and adolescent mental health service – a team of professionals specially trained to work with young people. They include child and adolescent psychiatrists . . . , psychologists, social workers, psychotherapists and specialist nurses.

From the Royal College of Psychiatrists website (www.rcpsych.ac.uk)

> ### Over to you
>
> The information above is taken from a booklet designed to enable children and adolescents to cope with stress. Identify some of the barriers it attempts to help them overcome and some of the benefits it identifies.

Conclusions

The bodily stress response is mediated by both neural and hormonal processes. The sympathetic adrenal medullary system responds quickly to immediate threats while the hypothalamic–pituitary–adrenocortical axis maintains a prolonged response to chronic stressors. This stress response is caused by a range of factors, both internal, such as our own thoughts or pain, and external, such as pressures of work or crowds. Biological factors such as the disruption of body rhythms, for example by shift work, and personality type may increase our susceptibility to the effects of stress. These factors can interact, compounding the effects on our ability to cope.

The effects of stress on the immune system are indirect. Although short-term stress may enhance our immune response, in the long term stress induces immunosuppression. As a consequence, chronic stress increases the risk of succumbing to infections and cancer. Psychoneuroimmunology investigates the link between stress, immunity and disease. In addition to this direct effect there are other consequences of stress, on health performance and social behaviour. Stressed people may suffer cardiovascular and gastrointestinal disorders, have poorer concentration and are more aggressive and less helpful.

People may use emotion- or problem-focused strategies to deal with stress, the latter being more effective but not always possible. Social support and educational resources can help people to resist the negative effects of stress.

> ### Over to you
>
> Find some different sources of information on dealing with stress, you might try in your doctors' surgery, at a local counselling service and on the Internet. Critically consider the advice given in the documents. Can you decide what strategies are being recommended? Justify the advice offered on the basis of the empirical evidence available to support each strategy.

RRRRR*Rapid recap*

Check your progress so far by working through each of the following questions.

1. Describe the three stages of the general adaptation syndrome.

2. Why might people with type A personalities be at greater risk from stress?

3. a. What is meant by emotion-focused and problem-focused coping strategies?

   b. Which coping strategies, emotion-focused or problem-focused, are more effective in general?

   c. In what situations would emotion-focused strategies be more beneficial than problem-focused ones?

If you have difficulty with more than one of the questions, read through the section again to refresh your understanding before moving on.

Key references

Other references are in the main reference list at the end of the book.

Carter, A.J. and West, M.A. (1999) Sharing the load: teamwork in health care settings. In: *Stress in Health Care Professionals* (eds R.L. Payne and J. Firth-Cozens). John Wiley, Chichester, pp. 191–120.

Evans, P. (1998) Stress and coping. In: *The Psychology of Health: An introduction* (eds M. Pitts and K. Phillips). Routledge, London, pp. 47–67.

Firth-Cozens, J. (1997) Predicting stress in general practitioners: 10 year follow up postal survey. *British Medical Journal*, **315**: 34–35.

Folkman, S., Larazus, R.S., Gruen, R.J. and DeLongis, A. (1986) Appraisal, coping, health status and psychological symptoms. *Journal of Personality and Social Psychology*, **50**: 571–579.

Langer, E.J. and Rodin, J. (1976) The effects of choice and enhanced personal responsibility for the aged: a field experiment in an institutional setting. *Journal of Personality and Social Psychology*, **34**: 191–198.

Stroebe, W. (2000) *Social Psychology and Health*. Open University Press, Buckingham.

Taffinder, N.J., McManus, I.C., Gul, Y. *et al.* (1998) Effect of sleep deprivation on surgeons' dexterity on laparoscopy simulator. *Lancet*, **352**: 1191.

5 Pain

An important role of health care professionals is to attempt to limit the suffering of their patients. Traditionally, in western medicine, this is achieved using drugs. However, as will become apparent in this chapter, there are other possible solutions to patient pain and patients themselves have a range of strategies that help them to cope with the pain they experience. An understanding of the nature of pain, factors that affect the patient's perception and the resulting pain behaviours will give you an insight into patients' experiences. A consideration of the ways in which pain can be managed, both professionally and by patients themselves, will enable you to support patients more effectively.

The nature of pain

Pain is one of the most intense feelings we can experience, yet our memory for it is oddly poor. We do, however, have a rich variety of words to describe the various forms of pain we can feel. There are dull aches, stabbing pains, 'hot' and 'cold' pains and pains that are mild, excruciating, nagging, burning, crushing, sickening or twisting. Clearly it is important, but what is it? It is related to physical harm – banging your head hurts – but it seems to be a lot more than just a simple reaction to injury. Pain has been defined as 'an unpleasant sensory and emotional experience associated with actual or potential tissue damage, or as described in terms of such damage' (International Association for the Study of Pain Subcommittee on Taxonomy 1979). In other words, pain hurts, physically and mentally, and arises when the body has been damaged or feels as though it has.

This definition allows us to identify several different facets of the experience. Pain is:

- A **neural** message that reaches the brain, so that we are aware of it

 Keywords

Neural
Relating to neurones or the nervous system

- Unpleasant, so it acts as a warning about or indication of damage to the body (although not all pain is 'useful', as some is unrelated to damage)
- Related to our senses, as it can be felt through any of them yet is different in nature from our ordinary sensations
- Affected by psychological as well as physical factors – a stimulus that is painful in one context may not be in another.

This definition does, however, assume that all pain is of peripheral origin, although evidence exists that some pain is psychogenic, i.e. it originates within the brain itself.

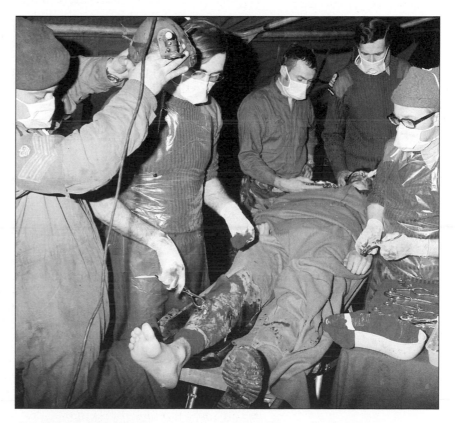

Our experience of pain depends on psychological factors. Beecher (1956) reported that soldiers who were badly injured in battle suffered considerably less pain than civilians with similar injuries. Think about how much your toe seems to hurt if you stub it when alone in the house or when you are with someone you want to impress with your bravery!

It is therefore possible to consider different 'dimensions' of pain. Four have been identified by Loeser (1989). These are:

- **Nociception** – the detection of tissue damage (a sensory experience)

Keywords

Somatosensory cortex
A band of tissue lying at the surface of the brain (the cortex) and running approximately across the top of the head (where a hair band would lie) that maps out sensation over the surface of our whole body, with proportionally more space allocated to those bodily areas with the greatest touch sensitivity, such as the hands and face, and in which adjacent body parts are aligned on the map

- **Pain** – the perception of that damage (interpreting the sensation)
- **Suffering** – the extent of distress (how much it hurts)
- **Pain behaviour** – the action taken that indicates tissue damage (both effective, such as putting a burn in cold water, or ineffective, such as swearing).

This classification is useful because it allows us to separate aspects of the pain experience and recognise that they may be independent of each other. We may have extensive tissue damage but not suffer, for instance if we are anaesthetised. In other situations we may have relatively less damage but experience more pain than in a different context, as Beecher found with civilians compared to soldiers (see photo on page 169). It is even possible to experience intense pain that appears to originate from a limb that has been amputated, as is the case for some patients with a 'phantom limb'. It is important, therefore, to recognise that patients may differ considerably in their experience of pain even when they have apparently identical physical conditions.

Phantom limb

Most people with amputations experience the sensation of a phantom limb and, for as many as 80% of them, this is accompanied by pain (Sherman *et al.* 1997). Traditionally, this has been explained as the consequence of activity in the sensory nerves that still exist between the point of amputation and the central nervous system (CNS) and that would, prior to amputation, have carried sensory messages from the limb. Cut nerves tend to form neuromas (nodules), which were believed to be the source of these signals, and treatment has been to sever the connection between the neuroma and the CNS. For some patients this relieves the pain, but in many it returns.

Evidence suggests, however, that the phantom limb sensation originates not in the extremities, but in the CNS itself, in a region called the **somatosensory cortex** (see also page 177). This consists of a sensory map of the body in which adjacent body parts are aligned on the map.

As neurones are capable of being reorganised to take over different roles, it has been suggested that phantom limb sensations may arise when the area of the somatosensory cortex apportioned to the missing limb becomes responsive to stimulation of some other part of the body, a process called remapping. This idea is supported by evidence from studies in which stimulation of adjoining parts of the body (such as regions of the face) produce precisely localisable sensations of touch in the phantom limb. Ramachandran (1993) described a patient in whom touching the face with a cotton bud produced matched sensations on the missing hand in the following pattern:

- Upper lip – index finger
- Lower lip – little finger
- Cheek – thumb.

This finding, and the absence of relief achievable by surgical means, strongly suggests that the phantom limb sensation is the result of remapping in the brain.

○━┱ *Keywords*

Priming
Preparing the body to expect a
specific stimulus

Melzack (1973) suggested that several factors might influence our perception of pain. These include attention, suggestion (**priming** that suggests we will or will not experience pain), anxiety, depression, learning (e.g. being conditioned to anticipate pain) and cultural expectations. This range of factors also suggests that there may be at least two aspects to the pain experience, since it has both a sensory component (e.g. where the pain is or what it feels like) and a psychological one (through which these influences could act). On page 178 we will begin to consider how these joint effects may be explained.

ᴙₑₜₗₑᴙ*Reflective activity*

If you have had the opportunity to observe or interact with more than one patient with the same physical damage (such as postoperative pain from identical surgery) consider what factors, other than the physical sensation from the site itself, could cause differences in the experience of pain for those individuals. Think also about the extent to which these patients have differed in their requests for analgesia.

Techniques for measuring pain

In order to begin to explore the various aspects of pain, researchers need to be able to measure people's experience of pain. This can be done in a number of different ways, some approaches focusing on the physical experience, others on the emotional component.

The self-report is a technique used both in research and in the context of health care, where nurses must assess patients' pain in order to collect information needed to make clinical judgements about the need for treatment. The individual describes his or her own experience, often using a chart to record the site and intensity of pain. Any pain relief administered may also be recorded here.

An alternative way to assess pain that has been used in clinical settings is based on psychophysics. This is a branch of psychology that aims to apply techniques from physics to assess our experiences and makes use of a measurements called thresholds – the smallest stimulus that can be detected – such as the faintest noise we can hear. For staff working with patients, two pain intensities are useful: the pain threshold (the point at which the patient perceives pain) and the pain tolerance point (the level of pain at which the patient resists pain, e.g. by restricting the movement of a painful joint).

The difference between these two levels provides a third measure, the pain sensitivity range. This, combined with the drug request point (the pain intensity at which the patient asks for pain relief) can help to guide clinical decisions.

Techniques used in research

Throughout this section we will be considering the relative usefulness of different measures of pain. The following are useful terms for assessing tools that measure pain.

Reliability

A judgement as to whether a measure (e.g. of pain) produces similar results each time it is used in a similar situation – e.g. would a patient give the same answers if tested twice? An unreliable measure is not useful as it cannot be trusted. If two people observed a patient and one recorded behaviours such as frowning and wincing (indicating pain), but the other recorded the patient getting up to the toilet and feeding herself, they would come to different conclusions about the patient's pain and would not be reliable

Validity

A judgement as to whether a measure really does assess what it claims to – pain – rather than some other factor such as the tendency of the individual to appeal for sympathy, or fear of pain and consequent requests for analgesia. If two independent measures of pain in a patient, such as a questionnaire and an observation, report similar pain levels they are considered to be valid.

Subjectivity

Refers to the influence of a personally biased perspective. For example, an individual reporting their own experiences and opinions or a health care professional or family member describing the pain behaviours of someone they know very well would be expressing subjective views.

Objectivity

Refers to an independent perspective, one that does not have the self as a point of reference. A range of techniques help to maximise this, including 'blind' procedures (where the treatment condition of the person being observed is not known to the observer), standardised instructions (e.g. to instruct all users of a questionnaire in the same way) and physiological measures such as pulse rate.

Self-reports and questionnaires

Self-reports may be open-ended descriptions, such as some pain diaries, or they may be more structured – using a questionnaire design – consisting of predominantly closed questions for the patient to respond to (see page 17 for question styles). Open-ended self-reports tend to be very subjective and it is difficult to determine whether they are valid or reliable; another measure of pain may be needed to assess whether the reporting of pain is consistent and comparable to other indicators. As a result, questionnaires are more often used in research.

> ### Over to you
>
> Before reading any further, try recording in your own words a description of a recent bout of pain you have experienced. It could be backache, hitting your head or having a serious injury. Include information about the onset, intensity, duration and nature of the pain, as well as any impairment it led to and the actions you took (if any) to control it.

As you will have found if you have tried the activity above, describing your own pain is difficult, even when guided by the prompts you were given. When people are asked to provide a self-report of their pain they are generally given much more directive questions. These may include:

- **Rating scales** – for example to measure the intensity of pain; these may ask for a score (such as 1–5, 1 being the most intense), a mark on a line (e.g. from 'no pain' to 'unbearable pain') on which the distance along the line is measured, or may have descriptors (such as 'pain free', 'mild pain', 'moderate pain', 'intense pain', 'as severe as any pain experienced')
- **Diagrams of the body** – to allow the individual to identify the apparent source of the pain even if they cannot describe its location
- **Behavioural measures** – to assess the impact of pain on the individual's functioning, e.g. asking whether they can walk or climb stairs
- **Forced choice items** – such as lists of words that describe types of pain.

The first three of these allow the researcher to measure the intensity and whereabouts of the pain but only the last offers an indication of the type of pain that is being experienced.

⊙━π *Keywords*

Rating scales
Provide a way to measure a continuous variable that does not necessarily have actual numerical values. They enable researchers to compare an individual's response from one occasion to another (e.g. whether the level of pain after treatment is less or more than before) but do not give a good indication of absolute levels of the variable

The most extensively used measure is the McGill Pain Questionnaire (Melzack 1975). It uses diagrams and forced-choice items, i.e. closed questions where the patient must choose only one descriptor of their pain, and provides an opportunity for an open response. It aims to assess three key facets of pain:

- **Evaluative** – cognitive judgements about the intrusiveness of the pain (e.g. troublesome, intense, unbearable)
- **Sensory** – a description of the nature of the pain (e.g. quivering, throbbing, pounding)
- **Affective** – the emotional component of the pain (e.g. punishing, gruelling).

Although the McGill Pain Questionnaire is considered to be both valid and reliable (e.g. Karoly 1985), it is not infallible. It does not distinguish well between different types of pain and is limited by the different, and subjective, way in which we use language – people may be unable to find a word that satisfactorily describes their particular pain or may want to choose two words from one category.

Clearly, the second part of the McGill Pain Questionnaire requires a good command of language, which not all patients, particularly children, necessarily have. In order to assess pain in children, Varni *et al.* (1987) developed a variation of the Questionnaire that asks children to use different colours to indicate the intensity of pain in different parts of the body.

Interviews

One important advantage of interviews over questionnaires is that, because the interviewer is listening to the patient's responses, he or she can alter the direction of questions if necessary. In a semi-structured interview the basic line of questioning is fixed but the interviewer can use his or her discretion, enabling the collection of useful information that might otherwise be missed. The product, however – a transcript of what was said – takes time and skill to use effectively.

Both self-reports (whether questionnaires or interviews) and observations can be unreliable. Patients may present aspects of their behaviour that they want to be acknowledged – for example, that they have difficulty moving or sitting if they want to take time off work. Alternatively, where closed questions are used, these may not allow patients to express themselves fully and symptoms may be overlooked. In observations, the observers may be biased – we tend to see what we expect to see – so a patient whom we believe to be recovering but who is struggling to conform to expectations may be judged to be in less pain than he or she is actually experiencing.

⚷ Keywords

Affective
In the context of psychology this refers to emotional components or feelings

As a result, we may choose to use a more objective measure – a physiological one.

Physiological measures

Pain is stressful, so some predictable stress-related changes could occur when we are in pain. These include changes in heart rate, sweating and muscle tension. Sweating can be assessed using galvanic skin resistance, a measure of the ability of the skin to conduct an electric current. When our skin is sweaty, and therefore watery, it conducts electricity better than when it is dry; as a result the resistance falls. Muscle tension can be measured with an electromyograph (EMG), an electrical record of the activity of muscles. If muscles are contracting abnormally, such as may be the case in lower back pain, this may be detected using an EMG. However, Wolf *et al.* (1982) found that in some patients suffering pain EMGs were elevated but in others they were reduced. The EMG may therefore be an unreliable indicator of pain.

A technique used in experimental pain research is the cold-pressor test. This induces pain by requiring the participant to immerse one hand first in water at room temperature then into water at 2°C. The participant's pain endurance is measured by the time they tolerate the cold water before removing their hand. Even though we can be certain that the participant is experiencing pain, and that it is likely to be similar from one occasion to another (i.e. reliable) we cannot be sure that the participant has actually reached their pain threshold when they choose to withdraw their hand. People can, of course, withdraw sooner, indicating a lower threshold than they actually have, thus invalidating the test.

The use of measures such as galvanic skin resistance and the cold-pressor test is, however, less helpful than you might expect. Precisely because the perception of pain has a psychological component, physiological indicators may not correlate well with the actual experience of suffering – as was shown with the EMG – hence they are not necessarily valid.

Observations

As observations can be made by someone other than the patient, they are more objective precisely because their source is not the sufferer. They may also be used when self-reports are judged to be unreliable, such as with children or people with **cognitive deficits** (e.g. stroke patients). The observer may look for:

- Indicators of the patient's functioning, such as activities of daily living or attendance at work or school

○━π Keywords

Cognitive deficits
Problems with attention, thinking, reasoning or memory

- Pain behaviours, such as crying or groaning, facial expressions, muscle tension or limping
- Requests for pain relief.

Observations may be conducted by trained professionals or **significant others**. Turk *et al.* (1983) have devised and used a system for spouses to record the effect of their partner's pain on behaviours such as work, recreation and family relations. This records when and where pain arises and allows for comparison with the patient's own assessment of their pain, facilitating some verification.

Professionals trained to observe pain behaviours use both 'covert' (hidden) but direct observations and indirect observations (e.g. using video). For example, Keefe and Block (1982) videotaped patients suffering lower back pain using two independent, trained observers. Their results were highly reliable – they tended to record similar frequencies of behaviours such as the patients sighing and rubbing or bracing themselves. In general, these related well to the patients' own reports of their pain, suggesting that these measures are also valid.

However, pain behaviours are reinforced, so may be performed more frequently than the patient's experience of pain would dictate. For example, a person may groan for attention, limp to avoid having to lift things for themselves, remain off work in order to gain compensation, stay on painkillers because they are frightened to do without or simply persist with their behaviour unconsciously because it provides rewards such as sympathy. Thus, observations of such behaviours may be flawed because they overestimate the actual experience of pain.

Keywords

Significant others
People who are close to an individual, such as a partner or family member

Theories of pain

Theories of pain attempt to explain how our perception of pain arises. An effective theory should be able to account not only for how pain originates but also how a range of factors, both physical and psychological, affect pain perception. In addition, it should be capable of explaining how pain-related phenomena such as phantom limb and the **placebo** effect occur. Finally, it should offer insight into the management of patient pain.

The specificity theory of pain

Early models of pain, from Descartes onwards, suggested that pain signals are detected and conveyed along pathways of neurones

Keywords

Placebo
An inert (inactive) chemical or procedure that is administered to patients or experimental participants, who believe that it is an active treatment

dedicated to the function, i.e. that are specific to pain and are transmitted to a 'pain centre' in the brain. Furthermore, the volume of the information carried about a particular pain indicates its intensity. One such theory was the specificity theory of pain (Von Frey 1895).

This approach led, unsurprisingly, to the general belief that the experience of pain was an exclusively physical event (dependent simply on an automatic response to tissue damage) and research endeavoured to find specific pain receptors or nerves (clusters of neural fibres). This search, however, has not been entirely successful. Although some sensory receptors are limited to a single kind of stimulus, many are responsive to a range of stimuli, including pain. Take, for example, the photoreceptors in the eye that detect light; they additionally respond to pressure (a gentle movement of the eyeball through the eyelid of a closed eye will generate visual effects) and very bright light is painful. Similarly, we have sensory fibres in our skin that detect pressure, heat and cold, but each of these will also react to intense stimulation as pain. Melzack (1993) observes that, if pain emanated solely from specific pain receptors then the pain associated with phantom limbs should not exist (see page 170). Nor, by the same reasoning, should referred pain be such a consistent phenomenon.

⊶ Keywords

Visceral
Relating to internal organs

Referred pain

The **somatosensory cortex** maps out superficial bodily sensation, apportioning more space to areas with greater sensitivity. As a consequence, we can pinpoint 'external' or superficial pain very accurately. However, there is no equivalent 'map' of our internal organs, so we are relatively poor at judging the exact source of **visceral** pain. Moreover, visceral pains are sometimes misinterpreted as superficial ones – we feel a pain caused by an internal problem as if it were 'on the outside'. This effect can be very reliable and thus has diagnostic value – patients complaining of a pain in the shoulder may be referred for cardiac investigations, as heart pain is often experienced in this way, as *referred pain*. In other words, it is generated in a region that is relatively pain-insensitive but is manifested as pain in an area with a greater density of pain receptors.

Evidence for the existence of pain fibres is also mixed: some authorities believe that fibres called 'A' and 'C' are exclusive to pain (e.g. Perl and Kruger 1996); others suggest they are not (e.g. Wall and Jones 1991). It seems unlikely that pain fibres are the only mechanism for providing information about pain, since, if they were, it would be possible to sever them and eliminate pain – but it is not.

Another problem for specificity theory is the failure of drugs to work on long-term pain. Whilst analgesics are effective for acute pain, such as a headache, they are much less successful at treating long-term pain (such as chronic backache). This suggests that tissue damage is not the only factor determining the intensity of pain.

As a consequence of the lack of evidence for the specificity theory and its inability to explain the variation in pain experienced with similar physical injuries (such as is demonstrated with soldiers, see page 169), we must conclude that it is at best incomplete as an explanation of pain. The most significant omission is its inability to explain the psychological influences on our experience of pain and failure to provide effective solutions for pain relief.

The gate control theory of pain

The most viable alternative to the specificity theory is the gate control theory of pain. This essentially suggests that, although pain messages may originate as sensory signals, these undergo several stages of modulation and interpretation, thus offering a route through which psychological variables could influence pain perception. Melzack and Wall (1965, 1982) proposed the theory, suggesting that pain signals from the body are channelled through a 'gate' in the spinal cord. If this gate is open, the individual experiences pain, but this message could be modulated – i.e. adjusted up or down – altering the pain perceived. The opening and closing of the gate, Melzack and Wall proposed, is governed by a range of factors, both physiological and psychological, since it receives not only physical signals from the body but also information from the brain (such as memories about previous pain, attention to the pain or emotions such as fear).

Reflective activity

Think about incidents where you have been in pain (perhaps you had twisted your ankle or developed a sore throat) then something happened to 'take your mind off it' – a phone call, you hit your funny bone or became engrossed in a good book. What happened to the pain?

Factors that close the gate (so reduce the experience of pain) include:

- **Physical factors** – analgesic drugs, stimulation of 'large' (A-beta) nerve fibres (e.g. by rubbing or scratching the skin), electrical stimulation of part of the midbrain area

- **Emotional factors** – relaxation, rest, optimism, happiness, excitement
- **Behavioural and cognitive factors** – distraction, concentration, knowledge that the pain will recede.

Factors that open the gate (so increase the experience of pain) include:

- **Physical factors** – physical damage, stimulation of 'small' (A-delta) and C nerve fibres
- **Emotional factors** – anxiety, pessimism, depression
- **Behavioural and cognitive factors** – focusing on the source of the pain, expecting to suffer pain.

In terms of explaining observations about the nature of pain, the gate control theory is clearly more successful than earlier models as it can account for the role of both physical and psychological

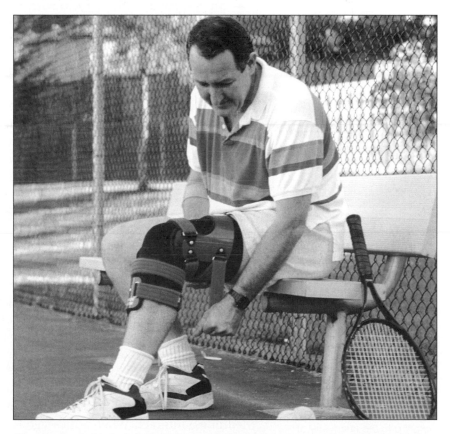

Signals about physical damage from an injury pass to the spinal cord and open the gate. However, psychological factors such as the lure of winning, being focused on the game and the cheering of onlookers counter this response and close the gate so the game goes on.

influences. It can also explain differing responses to painful situations, such as when we suck or rub a cut finger – the physical sensation closes the gate – but we can be unaware that we are badly hurt when focused on rescuing others from a crashed vehicle. Here, the psychological process of attention closes the gate and so prevents pain perception. As a consequence, the theory indicates routes to effective pain relief.

Over to you

Use gate control theory to explain each of the following experiences:
- Why adults insist on a 'rub-it-better' approach to childhood injuries – and it seems to work!
- Why, in the absence of any difference in the physical nature of an injury, it hurts more when we are relaxing at home in the evening than during a busy day at work
- Why a pain in the chest that you believed to be a heart attack might hurt more than an identical one you believed was indigestion
- How having a massage could reduce a headache
- Why sexual intercourse might decrease the experience of pain.

The exact physiological nature of the gate is, however, still unknown, although there is now evidence for physical mechanisms by which it may be opened and closed, for example the existence of opioids – naturally occurring molecules that opiate drugs resemble – which modulate the experience of pain. This, and other evidence accrued after the gate control theory was proposed, support the principle of a mechanism by which central (brain) processes can increase or decrease the perception of pain.

Endogenous opioids

Opiate drugs are those **psychopharmacological substances** that are extracted from the opium poppy or have a chemical structure similar to such compounds. The opiates include morphine, diamorphine hydrochloride, pethidine, codeine and many others; among them are some of the most powerful painkillers available. How do they work?

In order to understand the action of opiate drugs, we need to consider the **biochemical** activity that occurs when nerve cells (neurones) interact. When a message is passed from one neurone to the next it is a chemical signal, conveyed by small molecules called neurotransmitters. These are released from one neurone, travel across the gap between the cells (called the synapse) and attach to

Keywords

Endogenous
Formed within, e.g. endogenous opioids are formed (naturally) within the body

Psychopharmacological substances
Chemical substances that affect the brain

Biochemical
Relating to the chemistry of living things, such as the human body

specific locations on the membrane of the next neurone called receptor sites. Opiates, in common with many classes of drugs, act by mimicking naturally occurring neurotransmitter molecules, fitting into the receptor sites for a particular class of neurotransmitter. The drugs, and often the receptor sites, were discovered before the naturally occurring molecules themselves. The natural molecules thus derive their name from the drug group.

In the case of opiate drugs, the receptor sites are intended to receive molecules from a group called the endogenous opioids (think 'internal opiates') that were discovered in the 1970s (Pert and Snyder 1973). The endogenous opioids include the enkephalins and dynorphin – a molecule that is 200 times more effective than morphine at relieving pain. It seems that the opiate drugs function as analgesics because they mimic the body's own system for limiting pain. Pert has gone on to show that the **endorphins**, the molecules she had discovered, are also involved in functions known to relate to pain, such as emotions and the immune system (Pert *et al.* 1998).

Keywords

Endorphins
Opiate-like chemical substances naturally produced by the brain and pituitary gland to alleviate pain

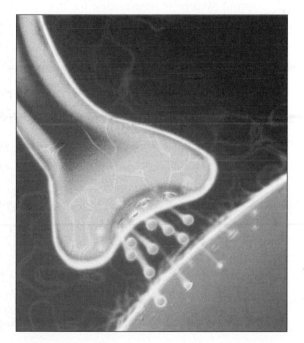

Communication between neurones is a chemical process. Neurotransmitter molecules cross the synapse and attach to receptor sites. These are the location of action for many drugs.

So, one of the roles of opioid molecules is to act as natural pain-suppressants in the body and research suggests that this action of opioids can be varied by a range of factors. Experiments investigating the effect of stress on pain perception in animals suggest that acute stress (such as in response to an electric shock) produces pain insensitivity, an effect called stress-induced analgesia. This suggests that psychological factors, such as stress, can trigger the release of endogenous opioids, thus reducing sensitivity to pain. Helmstetter and Bellgowan (1994) demonstrated stress-induced analgesia in rats in response to the stressor of noise. For one or two minutes after being exposed to a very loud noise, the rats were unresponsive to pain. They showed that this effect was the result of endogenous opiates by using naloxone, a drug that blocks the effect of both opiates and opioids by binding to their receptor sites. If the rats had been injected with naloxone prior to their exposure to the noise, no stress-induced analgesia occurred, demonstrating that stress-induced release of opioids must have been responsible for the initial pain-insensitivity of the rats.

Other factors that affect the release of endorphins include expectation, the timing and duration of painful stimuli, the individual's capacity to cope with the pain and their previous experience of pain (Sherman and Liebeskind 1980). The similarity of this list to that of the factors responsible for opening or closing the gate according to gate control theory is further evidence that the opioid system is responsible for implementing gate control. Furthermore, Sherman and Liebeskind (1980) have suggested that non-drug pain control methods may achieve analgesia by stimulating the release of endorphins (see also pages 183–185).

Acupuncture and endorphins

Acupuncture, used for centuries in China, claims to balance the two principles of nature, *yin* and *yang*, by correcting the 'lines of energy' (*qi*) believed to connect bodily structures. The technique uses long, thin needles inserted to differing depths at specific acupuncture points on the body, of which there are some 2000. The needles may be twirled, heated or electrically stimulated. Acupuncture has been traditionally used to treat a range of conditions such as headaches and arthritis. The practice continues, both in China and increasingly in other parts of the world, with considerable success.

Research suggests that acupuncture provides pain relief for some patients with a range of conditions. For instance, Coan *et al.* (1980) found that 83% of a group of back-pain patients receiving immediate acupuncture treatment improved, as did 75% of a delayed-treatment group. As with other treatments, it is important to distinguish the effects of the treatment from the effects of the patients' belief in the treatment, i.e. the placebo effect. To control for this, Vincent (1989) compared the effect of real acupuncture with a sham procedure and found that the effects of the real procedure on pain reduction were significantly greater, lasting more than a year post-treatment. Not all placebo studies have produced such promising results however (e.g. Dowson *et al.* 1985).

Brown (1972) reported that, since the 1960s, up to 90% of patients in China had undergone surgery with acupuncture, a procedure for which an electric current is passed between two or more needles. Acupuncture works for nearly everyone and the patient remains alert and interested (Melzack 1973). Analgesia through

continued

acupuncture takes time to build up and is maintained by a continuous current. The effect wears off slowly, although it can be prevented altogether by applying a local anaesthetic to the acupuncture points. These points are very specific, suggesting that acupuncture may operate on a principle akin to referred pain, but in reverse.

Some studies, such as that of Hui *et al.* (2000), have used imaging techniques to demonstrate the location in the brain of the effects of acupuncture on people in pain. The findings suggests that acupuncture-induced analgesia is mediated by the activation of descending pain messages, i.e. signals that close the gate, according to the gate control theory, thus reducing pain perception. This view is further supported by evidence from Chao *et al.* (1999), who showed that naloxone blocks the effect of acupuncture on blood pressure. Since naloxone reverses the effect of endogenous opioids (see page 184), this suggests that at least some of the effects of acupuncture must be mediated by endorphins.

(see page 184)

Keywords

Beta endorphin
A large endogenous opiate associated with the pituitary gland rather than the brain

Dysphoric
A state of psychological discomfort

Luteal and follicular stages
Refer to different stages of the menstrual cycle. During the follicular phase the ovaries produce oestrogen, which stimulates the growth of the lining of the uterus prior to ovulation. After ovulation, in the luteal phase, the hormone progesterone is secreted from the ovary and continues to prepare the uterus for fertilisation

In response to a painful stimulus, an area of the brain called the periaqueductal grey area is activated. This sends further messages through other brain areas and ultimately back down the spinal cord to the body. This route appears to modulate the pain signals, the inhibition resulting in a reduced perception of pain. If the periaqueductal grey area itself is electrically stimulated, a persistent and powerful analgesic effect is produced. Reynolds (1969) demonstrated that it was possible to perform surgery on laboratory animals using periaqueductal grey stimulation as the sole source of analgesia, and Basbaum and Fields (1984) have shown that direct injection of morphine into the periaqueductal grey produces significant pain relief even when it is used in minute quantities. This suggests that the periaqueductal grey is a key site at which opiates and opioids act. Further research has shown that the periaqueductal grey has a high density of opioid receptors and that it is stimulation of these that triggers the pain-relieving effect of the neural pathway leading down to the spinal cord.

Conversely, a lack of endogenous opioids may make some individuals more sensitive to pain than others. Straneva *et al.* (2002) measured pain sensitivity and **beta-endorphin** levels in women with premenstrual dysphoric syndrome. They found that these women, compared to controls, had lower pain thresholds, could tolerate pain for less time and rated pain as more unpleasant. Interestingly, the women with premenstrual **dysphoric** syndrome also exhibited lower beta-endorphin levels both in the **luteal and follicular stages** of the menstrual cycle, suggesting that their differing responses to painful stimuli might be determined physiologically.

Reflective activity

Think back to the ways in which patient pain, and that experienced by participants in pain research, would differ. In the light of gate control theory, how valid do you consider experimental studies of pain to be?

Endogenous opioids and the placebo effect

A placebo has been defined as 'any medical procedure that produces an effect in a patient because of its therapeutic intent and not its specific nature, whether chemical or physical' (Liberman 1962, p. 721). So, in the case of drugs, a placebo is an inert chemical that is administered to patients or experimental participants who believe that it is an active drug. Placebos are used in experimental situations in place of active drugs to control for any bias that may be created by the experience of being treated.

Placebos have been demonstrated to have analgesic effects and give symptom relief in conditions such as acne, allergies, asthma, cancer, diabetes, dementia, insomnia, multiple sclerosis and obesity (Haas *et al.* 1959). For example, Beecher (1959) injected patients suffering from pain with either morphine or a placebo. Those receiving morphine demonstrated significantly greater relief of pain, but the placebo did act as an effective analgesic in 35% of cases. Even sham operations (where the patients believe they have been operated on but no surgery has been completed) have been found to be as effective as real bypass operations at relieving the pain of angina (Diamond *et al.* 1960). In the alleviation of symptoms other than pain, however, placebo treatments do not appear to be effective (Hrobjartsson and Gotzche 2001). So, how could the analgesic effect of placebos arise?

Placebo treatment for dental pain – Levine *et al.* 1979

Aim: To investigate whether the placebo effect is related to endogenous opioids.

Procedure: Three hours after the extraction of a tooth, dental patients were given a placebo injection. After a further hour, the patients received an injection of naloxone (which blocks the effects of natural opioids, see page 182). Participants were given a baseline measure of sensitivity to pain and after each injection the participants rated their perception of pain on a standard scale.

Findings: The initial placebo injection reduced sensitivity to pain but the naloxone injection restored the participants' pain sensitivity.

Conclusion: The initial injection produced a placebo effect, however, this was abolished by the second injection suggesting that the placebo effect is mediated by the body's natural endorphins.

The findings of Levine *et al.* (1979; see box on page 184) suggest that the placebo effect may be mediated through the endorphin system. However, as we will see in the following sections, many psychological factors are involved in the extent of a placebo response.

Psychological factors affecting the perception of pain

We will now explore in a little more detail some of the psychological factors that appear to modulate the perception of pain.

Emotional factors

Anxiety

A patient's anxiety can affect their experience of pain. For example, Jamner and Tursky (1987) used exposure to pain-related words to make participants who were migraine sufferers more anxious. They found that the participants experienced more pain as a result. Similarly, McGowan *et al.* (1998) found a link between anxiety and the intensity of pelvic pain experienced by patients. However, according to Fordyce and Steger (1979), there is a difference between the role that anxiety plays in the control of acute versus chronic pain and this appears to be related to the efficacy – or otherwise – of drugs. An anxious patient suffering from acute pain is likely to obtain effective relief with the use of painkillers (simply because analgesia is more successful in the treatment of acute pain). The success of the treatment reduces anxiety and this contributes further to the reduction of pain (see right panel below). However, in the case of chronic pain, the failure of treatment can exacerbate anxiety, leading to greater fear and a more intense perception of pain (see left panel).

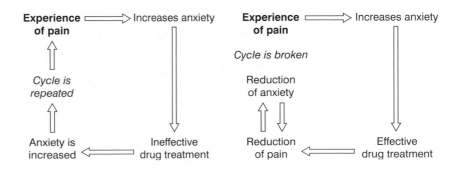

The effect of anxiety on the experience of acute and chronic pain

Behavioural factors

Learning plays a part in a patient's perception of pain. Individuals who have experienced pain before may have learned that pain, or pain relief, is associated with particular situations or behaviours.

Operant conditioning

In Chapter 2 we considered how learning theory could help us to understand ways to encourage people to acquire new health habits (page 55). The same explanation, of operant conditioning, can account for some variation in our experience of pain. Operant conditioning arises when an individual receives a reward (reinforcement) for performing a particular behaviour, and this results in them repeating that particular response. In the case of pain, people may receive reinforcement in the form of attention, sympathy or days off work as a result of exhibiting pain behaviours (such as groaning, resting or limping). However, as a consequence of the response they receive from others, their perception of the pain may actually increase (since these comments may serve to draw the individual's attention to their pain).

Classical conditioning

Another theory of learning is classical conditioning; this suggests that we acquire associations between stimuli when they occur together. If one stimulus spontaneously produces a response (such as a needle penetrating flesh producing pain and fear), one that is associated with it (such as the sight of a needle or being in a waiting room) may also begin to generate that response. As a consequence, people may learn that injections are painful, so become nervous in the waiting room or if they see a syringe.

Apart from the conditioned response, two other factors are at work here. One is expectation – the individual is anticipating pain, which, terms of the gate control theory, opens the gate. In addition, the patient may become anxious – their anxiety will also open the gate. Therefore classical conditioning can help to explain how experience may lead to increased perception of pain.

Conversely, the same process may explain the placebo effect. Since we tend to experience symptom reduction in association with taking medication, the response of pain relief is acquired to the stimulus of seeing and swallowing tablets. Since repeated exposure to this pairing of the drug as a stimulus and pain relief as a response results in classical conditioning, eventually the act of swallowing tablets that appear to be a drug will result in the same response. This arises in much the same way as a dog learns to salivate because it sees a tin of food being opened – the tin and the food are normally associated so eventually even the tin, in the absence of any food, can cause salivation. Such classically conditioned associations could also account for the placebo effect (see box below).

Classical conditioning

Dog food	→	Salivation
Dog food + dog food tin	→	Salivation
Dog food tin	→	Salivation
Pain of injection	→	Fear
Pain of injection + seeing needle	→	Fear
Needle	→	Fear
Taking (real) tablets	→	Pain reduction (due to tablets)
Seeing and taking tablets	→	Pain reduction (due to tablets)
Seeing and taking (placebo) tablets	→	Pain reduction (due to conditioning)

Cognitive factors

Expectancy

Expectancy refers to the influence that our beliefs about possible outcomes have on our experience. If we have faith in a particular consequence or effect, then this is more likely to arise.

Expectancy and the placebo effect

The placebo effect was described earlier (page 184) in relation to the role of endogenous opioids. We will now consider how psychological factors, rather than physiological ones, might play a part in this phenomenon. In an experiment investigating the effects of placebos, Gefland *et al.* (1963) manipulated participants' beliefs by giving them a drug reputed to be an analgesic. These participants experienced greater pain relief than control participants who received no treatment.

In a review of several placebo studies, De Craen *et al.* (1996) reported on the relative effectiveness of placebos of different colours. Actual analgesics were equally effective regardless of colour but, whilst participants taking blue and green 'painkiller' placebos did experience some analgesic effects, the red placebos were as effective as the actual drugs. Similarly, bigger placebo pills are more effective than smaller ones (Berg 1977). At a psychological level, it can be argued that placebo effects such as these, whether mediated by endogenous opioids or not, are a consequence of the patient's expectations; the belief that a procedure will be effective plays some part in its success. This explanation is not necessarily in conflict with a physiological one, since expectations could initiate the central nervous system activity that triggers endorphin release.

Varied sources of evidence suggest that expectations are important in the placebo effect. These include:

- Greater placebo efficacy if they appear to be genuine medication, for example if they look like drugs and are given to the patient in a medical setting (Shapiro 1964)
- Greater placebo efficacy when they are administered by confident, high-status health care practitioners (Shapiro 1964)
- The capacity of placebos to generate side effects (commonly headaches and nausea) if these are expected by patients, in addition to alleviating symptoms (Gowdey 1983)
- Similar effects of dosage, latency and strength of the placebo in comparison to actual medication (Ross and Olson 1981)
- Placebo treatments with technological-sounding names are effective (e.g. 'subconscious reconditioning', Lent *et al.* 1981).

These findings all suggest that patients' prior knowledge about actual medication affects the outcome of a placebo trial – a foul-tasting tablet that requires a regular regime, prescribed with confidence in a medical context will be highly effective.

these taste like pond water and are almost impossible to swallow – they'll cure me in no time!

In a study similar to the one described in the box on page 185, Gracely *et al.* (1985) investigated the effect of practitioner expectations on the effectiveness of a placebo. Patients having a wisdom tooth extracted were injected with either:

- Fentanyl (an analgesic)
- Naloxone (which reverses the effects of endogenous opiates)
- A placebo.

They were told that the injection might reduce or increase their pain or have no effect. There were two categories of patient: some could receive any of the injections, others only either naloxone or the placebo. The practitioners knew whether patients were in the three- or two-option group but were unaware of their exact treatment. Interestingly, the doctors' expectations had an effect. Only those patients whom the practitioners believed could receive painkillers (i.e. those in the first group) experienced pain reduction. Since the patients did not know which group they were in, the only possible explanation is that practitioners' beliefs resulted in the appearance of the placebo effect when there was a possibility of actual pain relief but the absence of such an effect when there was no chance of receiving analgesics.

One source of patients' beliefs is the opinion of their practitioner; hence we would expect this to affect expectancy. The influence of apparent practitioner belief on the placebo effect was illustrated in a study conducted by Park and Covi (1965). Fifteen patients were told that their condition was often helped by sugar pills and that these contained no medication. Fourteen of the patients volunteered to try the sugar pills, of whom 13 experienced significant clinical improvement. The practitioner effects were sufficiently great to act as a placebo even when the patients were aware that their medication contained only sugar.

Practitioner effects such as those described above can also operate in reverse. Feldman (1956) showed that the efficacy of the tranquilliser chlorpromazine reduced from a typical 77% success to only 10% when it was prescribed by a practitioner who expressed doubts about its capacity to reduce symptoms. This provides further evidence to suggest that patient expectations can affect symptoms directly.

Key points Top tips

Placebo effects may be mediated by a combination of factors, including:

- **Physiological factors** – the release of endogenous opioids such as endorphins
- **Patient expectations** – belief in the treatment increases the efficacy of treatment
- **Practitioner expectations** – expressed confidence in the treatment enhances the placebo effect
- **Classical conditioning** – the patient's previous encounters with treatments that have resulted in symptom reduction will have built up an association between taking medication and pain relief.

Expectancy and the perception of pain

Just as a patient's expectations may affect their response to a placebo, they may also affect the perception of pain itself. A patient who is anticipating pain is more likely to experience it. As we saw in the section on anxiety (page 185), the prospect of enduring pain or a painful procedure tends to increase the patient's suffering. This is also illustrated by cultural differences in requests for pain relief.

For example, women from different cultural backgrounds have differing expectations about the pain they will experience during childbirth (Streltzer 1997). As a consequence, they differ in their apparent experience of pain and their strategies for coping. The cultural norm for Yap women in the south Pacific is for childbirth to be part of day-to-day life, so pregnant women continue with their normal routine until the moment of birth and return to an active life after a short rest. This expectation of ease may account in part for the low incidence of complications (Kroeber 1948). In contrast, Mexican women are primed to expect childbirth to be painful, as their word for labour, *dolor*, means 'pain' or 'sorrow'. This expectation and fear of the birth process compound to result in more painful experiences (Scrimshaw *et al.* 1983).

Cultural differences are also found in the pain relief offered to patients with cancer. In China, only about 4% of cancer patients receive opiate drugs, whereas the figure is closer to 70% in Europe. These patterns may be partly accounted for by differences in health care between countries. However, evidence from Ng *et al.* (1996) suggests that within the USA differences exist between the postoperative pain relief given to patients from different ethnic groups. White Americans receive more analgesia postoperatively than do African or Hispanic Americans.

Cognitive dissonance

Recall the sensation when you've bought something that maybe you shouldn't have – a new CD or a pair of shoes. You then engage in an internal process of justification – it might go along the lines of 'it's better quality/more unusual than this alternative'. The conflict that you feel is the consequence of cognitive dissonance. Festinger (1957) proposed the theory of cognitive dissonance to account for our tendency to make decisions that minimise our experience of tension because we need to:

- Justify our behaviour
- Perceive ourselves to be rational and in control.

So, according to Festinger, we debate the doubtful purchase, justifying it with thoughts like 'it was a bargain' to overcome our dilemma, allowing us to perceive the action to have been a rational one.

Cognitive dissonance and the placebo effect

Cognitive dissonance theory has been used to account for the placebo effect (Totman 1976, 1987). It suggests that, precisely because we are prepared to make sacrifices – such as drinking revolting medicine or enduring the pain of an injection – there must be a concomitant benefit, namely an improvement in our condition. In fact, we make many 'investments' in our health, not least the payment of taxes or health insurance to fund our health care. In addition, we are likely to have spent time and effort seeing a doctor, as well as costs such as travelling or taking time off work.

These investments can only be justified if we experience a gain; without any apparent benefit we would feel stupid, cheated or misled. So we justify our behaviour by believing that the treatment works and thus avoid the feeling of dissonance created by perceiving ourselves to have been irrational. There is a 'choice', although not necessarily a conscious one. We could accept that there has been no change in our health but this requires us to accept that we have been duped – hence the dilemma.

When cognitive dissonance is applied to the placebo effect, we can see that individuals, be they research participants or patients, have a source of unconscious motivation for believing that they have experienced the desired effect from taking medication or receiving treatment. For real patients, these are the costs described above. For participants in experiments, the cost may have been the time and trouble spent engaging in the research, as well as any negative experiences associated with the placebo treatment. Furthermore, they need to believe that the research is worthwhile – that the proposed new treatment 'works' – otherwise they have wasted their effort. Thus, in order to avoid the discomfort of dissonance, individuals must justify their behaviour by identifying positive outcomes such as pain reduction.

However, neither in the case of research participants nor real patients can we be sure that cognitive dissonance is adequate as an explanation. Since it depends on unconscious mechanisms (the internal dilemma and a need to 'solve' it) we would need to independently demonstrate their existence to be certain.

Some evidence comes from research that demonstrates the importance of justification. Totman (1987) conducted an experiment in which pain was caused to participants (using heat stimulation), who were then told they were receiving an analgesic that was in fact a placebo. Some of these participants were put in a state of low need for justification by giving them a payment for participation – they could therefore justify to themselves any pain they suffered on the basis of their financial reward, so would suffer little dissonance – their behaviour 'made sense'. 'High need for justification' participants received no payment and, according to cognitive dissonance theory, would require greater justification from the experimental setting in order to avoid experiencing the dissonance associated with behaving irrationally – having suffered pain for no reason.

Totman's findings were as predicted – the high justification group reported less pain than the low justification group, suggesting that a need to justify one's behaviour can cause a placebo effect. We cannot be sure, however, whether people in such situations are genuinely experiencing reduced pain or simply reporting it less – since this could also serve to reduce dissonance. Nevertheless, this theory offers a plausible explanation for placebo effects, not just with regard to pain reduction but also the relief of other symptoms using placebo treatments.

Coping with pain

It is worth beginning this section with an observation from Krokosky and Reardon (1989) that health care professionals (including doctors and nurses) tend to underestimate the amount and duration of pain suffered by patients. This is problematic, since the role of health care professionals is to reduce suffering and it is generally accepted that it is easier to keep pain at bay than to allow it to become intense before attempting to gain control.

There are a number of different ways that pain can be controlled to the extent that a patient can cope. These include:

● removing the patient's sensory capacity so that they feel nothing at all from the affected area, i.e. anaesthesia – the loss of sensation

● removing the patient's capacity to feel pain in the affected area, although they may still be aware of a sensation, i.e. analgesia – the numbing of pain without loss of consciousness

● altering the patient's perception of the sensation such that, although it is still painful, they are no longer concerned – i.e. enabling them to cope by reducing their awareness

● altering the patient's capacity to tolerate the pain so that, although it is still as painful, they are less debilitated by it – i.e. enabling them to cope by increasing their resistance.

Some pain control strategies clearly use only one of the above processes; for example, a nerve block administered spinally prevents the detection of any sensation. Other strategies, however, employ a mixture of processes and it is not always possible to separate these.

So, the possible options open to patients and their health carers for coping with pain can be broadly categorised into physiological/ physical methods and psychological strategies. Some examples include:

● Physiological/physical control methods:
  – Drugs
  – Physical stimulation (e.g. counterstimulation, **transcutaneous electrical neurological stimulation – TENS**)
  – Surgical procedures
● Psychological coping strategies:
  – Relaxation
  – Biofeedback
  – Hypnosis.

Traditionally, patient pain has been treated medically, with predominantly physiological and physical methods. However, as our understanding has changed, for example the insight that gate control theory has given to the role of psychological factors in the patient's perception of pain, this narrow view of pain management has given way to a broader approach that encompasses psychological strategies too.

We will look briefly at the physiological and physical methods of pain control and then consider some of the psychological strategies (relaxation, hypnosis and biofeedback) in detail, but first we will

⊶ₙ Keywords

Transcutaneous electrical neurological stimulation (TENS)

A system of electrical skin stimulation that is effective in reducing pain in some patients consider individual differences between patients' own strategies for coping.

Pain, locus of control and coping strategies

In addition to offering specific therapeutic approaches to pain control, psychological approaches can provide health care professionals with an insight into the independent resources that individuals have for coping with their own pain. So, before we explore how pain might be managed, we will look at two aspects of the individual patient that affect the way in which they view and attempt to deal with problems including pain.

Rotter (1966) described the concept of locus of control, a measure that describes the extent to which an individual perceives that they themselves, or some other, external force, is responsible for determining the course of events in their lives. The idea has been applied both to health and pain, using the health locus of control (Wallston *et al.* 1978) and the pain locus of control (Manning and Wright 1983). These measures assess the level of self-determination versus external causation an individual perceives with respect to their health or experience of pain (see also page 145). Essentially, it suggests that patients who attribute control to factors they cannot govern, such as luck or whether they have a good consultant, are described as having an external locus of control. Those who believe that they are responsible for actions that affect themselves, such as remembering to take their medication regularly have an internal locus of control. So, an individual's locus of control can clearly affect how actively they engage in their own pain management. In addition, it appears to have a bearing on their actual experience of pain.

Crisson and Keefe (1988) found that patients with an external pain locus of control felt that they were unable to exert control over their own experience of pain. Those with an internal locus of control, however, had fewer physical and psychological symptoms and responded better to treatment. Patients with an external locus of control may tend to 'catastrophise', i.e. imagine the worst, such as a failure to ever recover. Burton *et al.* (1995) showed that such patients were likely to suffer greater pain.

A second patient characteristic, also discussed in depth in Chapter 4, is the idea of coping strategies, i.e. the extent to which the individual employs emotion- or problem-focused strategies for dealing with a stressful situation such as being in pain. Where there are useful steps the patient can take to deal with their own pain, problem-focused strategies are beneficial. For example, when adhering to appropriate schedules of exercise, rest or pain-killers effectively limits pain, patients gain from being problem-focused. However, where there is little or nothing patients can do to minimise their suffering, as when an injured patient is awaiting surgery, emotion-focused strategies that allow them to ignore the problem or blame someone else will be more helpful.

Experimental evidence from Jackson *et al.* (1979) showed that participants exposed to inescapable pain (mild electric shocks), so they could only use emotion-focused strategies, experienced spontaneous endorphin-related pain relief. However, those exposed to escapable pain (i.e. they could take action to avoid the pain, employing a problem-focused strategy) did not. Affleck *et al.* (1992) investigated the effect of emotion-focused strategies (emotional support and distraction) on pain perception. They found them to be effective in reducing perceived pain when pain levels were low but they were ineffective for individuals with more intense pain.

Both of the above ideas are incorporated into the fear-avoidance model, which, in essence, suggests that, because individuals can experience pain sensations and behaviours separately, their perception of pain can become distorted. Importantly, it suggests that fear can enhance pain perception. As a consequence, it suggests that pain avoidance behaviours are counterproductive to recovery, so those individuals who confront pain are likely to make faster recoveries (Letham *et al.* 1983). In line with this prediction, Klenerman *et al.* (1995) found that back pain patients who showed fear-avoidance recovered more slowly.

The management of acute and chronic pain

As we have seen elsewhere in the chapter (page 185), acute and chronic pain present different problems in terms of management. Acute pain, by definition, is short-lived (lasting less than 6 months). This alone may be important for a patient's coping. The knowledge that physical recovery will lead to pain reduction is an important psychological component, as is optimism arising from seeing physical signs of tissue healing (such as removal of a plaster cast or reduced scarring). These are likely to be absent for a patient suffering from chronic pain. Another important difference is the efficacy of painkillers. Both placebo and actual drugs tend to be effective in the control of acute pain but ineffective against chronic pain.

Furthermore, the experience of chronic pain often leads to a constellation of symptoms and behaviours that are self-fulfilling. For example, patients in chronic pain may:

- **Be stressed** – this will exacerbate their pain

- **Have limited social or recreational opportunities** – this will reduce their social support and increase their attention to the pain, increasing their perception of it
- **Engage in pain behaviours**, such as complaining or avoidance, that may further limit social support, even from close relatives and partners
- **Take a range of medications with little or no efficacy** – they may, however, have side effects
- **Suffer from depression** – which may increase their perception of pain and decrease the possibility of effective self-management of pain.

The differences outlined above suggest that strategies for the management of acute and chronic pain may differ considerably.

Physiological and physical methods of pain control

Analgesic medication

Morphine, a highly effective painkiller (see page 180), is widely used in the control of acute pain, for example postoperatively and in the management of cancer pain. However, it has two significant disadvantages for patients who take it for a prolonged time: they may become dependent, and they may experience tolerance – i.e. a greater dose will be required to achieve the same analgesic effect. As a consequence, other drugs may be used in preference to morphine. However, concerns about the risk of developing dependence (becoming addicted) are greatly exaggerated. The number of patients who develop dependence to prescription medication following surgery is very small indeed (Porter and Jick 1980), whereas many patients with a legitimate need for analgesia are undermedicated as a consequence of such misplaced fears (Taylor 1995).

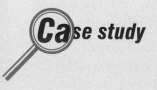 **Keywords**

Patient-controlled analgesia (PCA)

A system of administering a pain-killing drug intravenously in which the patient has control over the frequency of doses (up to a predetermined limit)

Case study

Eleanor – victim of undermedication

Eleanor, who was in hospital for routine abdominal surgery, was returned to her room after a prolonged period in the recovery room during which it had proved difficult to get her postoperative pain under control. During the following night, Eleanor, who was still using **patient-controlled analgesia (PCA)** with diamorphine, called a nurse, as the pain was worsening. The nurse removed the intravenous line completely, believing Eleanor to have become addicted in less than 18 hours and leaving her in considerable distress. The pain worsened during the following day and, although Eleanor had been seen by her consultant in the morning, he was recalled that afternoon. One glance at Eleanor's wound indicated that it had reopened and she would need to be readmitted for further surgery later that evening.

ɘ̃ʇɘЯ*Reflective activity*

- Was the removal of the intravenous line justified or appropriate?
- What effects, other than the significant increase in pain suffered by the patient, would have arisen from the removal of pain relief?

There are other, less addictive but also less powerful analgesics than the opiates. These include ibuprofen, paracetamol and aspirin. The exact mechanism of these analgesics is not, however, fully understood. A brief tabulation of analgesics and their properties is given in Table 5.1.

Table 5.1 Analgesics and their properties

Drug group	Examples	Mode of action	Disadvantages
Opiates	Morphine Diamorphine Pethidine Tramadol Codeine	Mimic endogenous opioids	Risk of dependence and tolerance with long-term use; short-term effects of constipation, poor judgement
	Aspirin	The active ingredient, acetylsalicylic acid, was the prototype non-steroidal anti-inflammatory drug (NSAID). It also reduces inflammation and lowers temperature in fever	Increases clotting time (problematic for patients with wounds); can cause gastric irritation; toxic in large quantities (causing liver and kidney damage)
	Paracetamol	Reduces temperature but has little anti-inflammatory effect	Toxic in relatively small quantities (causing kidney damage)
Other NSAIDs	Ibuprofen Diclofenac	Block synthesis of prostaglandins which are released at the site of damage or inflammation and sensitise pain-conducting neurones	Less effective on pain not associated with inflammation; can cause gastric irritation; toxic in large quantities (causing liver and kidney damage)

Two other techniques for drug-induced analgesia include nerve blocks and the use of antidepressants. Spinal blocks prevent the transmission of pain messages up the spinal cord, thereby preventing the perception of pain. These may be used as analgesia for surgery, for example Caesarean sections. Antidepressant drugs may also have analgesic properties and these are enhanced by the effect of anxiety reduction. As such, antidepressants may be effective in countering chronic pain.

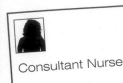
Consultant Nurse

Professionally speaking . . .

Pain management – a range of roles: An interprofessional approach

Pain management can involve a whole range of health care professionals, particularly pharmacists, doctors and specialist nurses. I had one patient on the ward with a cancerous mass and she was deteriorating quite quickly, and she was on oral morphine solution every 6 hours. We got the pain care specialist nurse to review her to see if having a syringe driver of diamorphine would be appropriate. Because as nurses we're there looking after patients all the time we have more indication of whether they're in pain and when to call in other health professionals. The registrar prescribed this, and she settled much better, and was not crying out when we tried to move her.

Physical stimulation as a control measure for pain

Counterstimulation is a pain control measure achieved by stimulating, or irritating, another part of the body. A possible explanation for the mechanism by which counterstimulation may work was discussed on page 178, in the context of the gate control theory.

Transcutaneous electrical nerve stimulation (TENS) is a system of electrical skin stimulation that is effective in reducing pain in some patients (Melzack and Wall 1982). Electrical stimulation from the electrodes penetrates to a depth of about 4 cm and the patient can control both the location of the electrodes and the frequency and strength of the electrical signals. When effective, relief following a session of TENS treatment can last for several hours and may be used to combat some instances of both acute and chronic pain.

Surgery as a control measure for pain

Surgical lesions to pain fibres prevent the transmission of pain signals from the body up to the brain. Such lesions may be made either in the peripheral nervous system or in the spinal cord. These procedures are an extreme solution and, although they may be successful in reducing pain, the benefits are often only short term. If the pain does return, it may be worse than before – due to the nerve damaged caused by the operation – and may even result in phantom-limb-type pain. In addition, the surgery itself carries risks and the possibility of side effects, as well as being expensive.
The pain probably returns because the nervous system, contrary to received wisdom, is now thought to have considerable capacity for regeneration, with neural pathways being re-routed through remaining nerves, thus restoring the severed connection.

Psychological strategies for coping with pain

Acupuncture, discussed on page 182, is sometimes regarded as a psychological technique for coping with pain. As research progresses, the physiological process by which the effects of acupuncture arise are becoming apparent.

In this section, three strategies that are more clearly psychological in nature are discussed: relaxation, biofeedback and hypnosis. However, it is important to bear in mind that these strategies, like acupuncture and the placebo effect, must have underlying physiological mechanisms and they may ultimately be uncovered.

Cognitive behavioural therapy

One psychological approach to pain management is the use of cognitive-behavioural strategies. This approach recognises the role of different sources of experience in pain perception and coping:

- **Thinking** – for example, what pain means to the individual 'I am in too much pain to continue with my job'
- **Emotions** – how the individual feels about their pain, for example 'I'm frightened that it won't ever get easier to bear'
- **Physiology** – the role of the nervous system, for instance impulses from a site of injury
- **Behaviour** – for instance avoiding exercise because it hurts.

As its name implies, cognitive behavioural therapy (CBT) employs a range of strategies to tackle both cognitive issues, including thoughts and beliefs that lead the patient to focus on the pain, and behaviour – changing the way a patient responds to their experience of pain. A cognitive behavioural therapist aims to increase the individual's self-control over their pain and uses intrinsic (internal) sources of reinforcement to sustain these changes. This aim may be achieved in a number of different ways, for example by reducing the attention the patient devotes to the pain or to change pain related behaviours and beliefs. Some specific goals of CBT may include:

- **Overcoming demoralisation** – feelings of helplessness can be restructured to allow individuals to see their pain as manageable
- **Reducing counterproductive strategies** – patients may have learned maladaptive coping strategies, such as avoiding exercise, that actually worsen their pain; CBT teaches them to be aware of such feelings and behaviours
- **Skills training** – adaptive strategies are taught so that the patient has alternative ways to cope; these may include

refocusing attention away from the pain, thus reducing the distress experienced.

- **Increasing self-efficacy** – passive patients are taught to accept that they have control and competence
- **Self-attribution** – patients may believe that success in treatment is attributable to others but that they are to blame if treatment fails; they are taught that they too can be responsible for positive outcomes
- **Encourage future coping** – patients are taught ways to anticipate problems and develop their own strategies to cope with them, so that the effects of the intervention are lasting
- **Belief in treatment efficacy** – patients with chronic pain whose treatments have been unsuccessful may believe that no treatments work; they are taught to believe that CBT will improve their condition.

Cognitive behavioural therapy has been successful in reducing pain and improving coping. For example, Thomas *et al.* (1999) found that CBT not only reduced pain and distress in patients with sickle-cell disease but also helped their ability to cope. This effect was evident both immediately after the intervention and at 2 months post-treatment. Similarly, Basler and Rehfisch (1990) used CBT for chronic pain sufferers with head, shoulder, arm or spine pain, who showed improvement compared to individuals in a control group. Immediately after following a 12-week CBT programme the patients reported benefits including lower intensity pain, less impairment, a more positive mood, better sleep and less anxiety and depression compared to the controls. Most of these gains (except mood and sleep problems) persisted to the 6-month follow-up, suggesting that CBT provides lasting benefits in terms of pain reduction and enhanced coping.

These changes appear to be the result of the intended changes in the patients' beliefs and self-efficacy. Dolce (1987) found that patients on a treatment programme who experienced reduced pain, but attributed this improvement to the therapist rather than to changes in their own skills, were less likely to continue to use the strategies they had learned and were more likely to relapse after the intervention.

Relaxation

Relaxation techniques were originally developed as a means to help clients with anxiety disorders such as phobias. Wolpe (1958) developed a technique known as systematic desensitisation in which relaxed clients progressively lose their fear of previously phobia-inducing situations such as small spaces or snakes. Since this technique works primarily by reducing anxiety, and this is one of the key psychological factors in increasing a patient's experience of pain, it follows that anxiety-reduction should be efficacious in pain control. In addition, for those sources of pain that are directly related to or exacerbated by physical tension, relaxation should also reduce pain.

Effective relaxation requires not only the reduction of tension in muscles but also a slowing of the breathing rate. During relaxation training initial deep breaths are followed by slower, deeper breaths than the client usually takes and they are more focused on the rhythm of their own breathing.

Holroyd and Penzien (1990) found that relaxation was more effective than a placebo in the treatment of recurrent migraine headaches. However, this treatment was more effective still if combined with biofeedback (see next section).

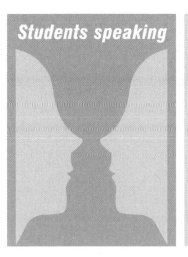

Students speaking

The importance of relaxation in symptom control is illustrated by this student's experience . . .

Research nurse

The one place where I saw the use of relaxation was in a group home for clients with learning disabilities. They had a 'relaxation therapy room' that had 'Austin Powers' psychedelic lights, throws and big, fluffy cushions. They used it for people with challenging behaviours, and when I was in there I felt that I could have floated away.

Biofeedback

Biofeedback is the use by patients of information about changes in their own condition to enhance their recovery. This feedback about biological status, such as temperature, blood pressure, heart rate or muscle tension, is provided to patients by giving them access to a standard physiological measure (such as skin temperature, blood pressure or heart rate monitors or electromyogram readings).

The process operates on a classical conditioning paradigm (discussed earlier on page 186). This learning mechanism suggests that biofeedback occurs because the stimulus – such as a tilt-table used to produce a desired effect of reducing blood pressure – becomes associated with the new stimulus of thinking about the effect. After

○━━🔑 *Keywords*

Raynaud's disease
A condition in which blood supply, particularly to the digits, is over sensitive to cold, causing circulation to the fingers and toes to fail

repeated pairings, classical conditioning results in the new stimulus, i.e. thinking about the effect, becoming capable of independently causing the desired response. This process has been used effectively to reduce pain in conditions such as **Raynaud's disease** (using feedback about skin temperature) and hypertension (using feedback about blood pressure). It is particularly useful as it allows patients to play a central role in their own symptom management and, furthermore, is effective with some chronic conditions.

However, despite the sound reasoning behind biofeedback, it appears that modification of the target process (such as lowering blood pressure) and reduction of pain are not necessarily related (Turk *et al.* 1979). For example, although some studies (e.g. Nakao *et al.* 1997, Paran *et al.* 1996) have found benefits to patients using biofeedback to reduce blood pressure, McGrady (1994) failed to demonstrate a lasting effect. Other influences, such as relaxation or the placebo effect, may in fact be responsible for the beneficial changes observed in biofeedback.

Hypnosis

Franz Anton Mesmer (hence the term 'mesmerised') was the first documented practitioner of what is now called hypnosis. He aimed to use his skills therapeutically and believed that the effects he induced in people were a result of his own 'magnetism'. Although Mesmer is unlikely to have been magnetic, his clinical practice was demonstrably effective. More recently, techniques of relaxation, eye fixation – focusing on an object and verbal cues such as feeling heaviness in the eyelids – or a sensation of moving downwards are used to induce a state of hypnosis. Effectively administered to a susceptible person, these procedures lead to a condition of relaxed suggestibility that can have useful clinical effects. The hypnotised patient will respond to suggestions of imagery made by the therapist and these may be used to provide a context within which the awareness of pain is limited.

Both analgesia and anaesthesia are possible through hypnosis. A measure of analgesia may arise spontaneously during hypnosis; as the subject becomes absorbed in the imagery, their awareness of other sensations diminishes. This is comparable to not realising we have gone numb from sitting still for hours reading a good book. A greater analgesic effect can be achieved by direct suggestion. This can result from suggested loss of sensation, e.g. as a 'glove' protecting the hand from pain, or by guiding the subject to feel separate from that part of the body. Other techniques use age progression or regression to take the client forwards or backwards in time to a pain-free age, and suggestions to 'forget' the pain (Yapko 1995).

Professionally speaking . . .

Hypnosis, CBT and the treatment of pain

Clinical psychologist

As a clinical psychologist using hypnosis I see clients with problems ranging from simple phobias to the long-term effects of childhood abuse. A significant proportion of my caseload, however, consists of people who have problems with pain or a fear of potentially painful procedures. With these I use hypnosis as a context for teaching cognitive behavioural pain management strategies such as sensory transformation, detachment and imaginative inattention, as well as using direct analgesia suggestions.

Sometimes these can be very short interventions. On a number of occasions I have been asked by clients to help them to cope with a forthcoming surgical procedure – often this request has come the day before their operation. My usual method for this is the so-called 'special place' technique, in which clients are taught in hypnosis to take themselves to a safe and relaxing place of their own choosing (warm, sunny beaches are very popular) where 'nothing can bother them'. After a single session of training they are then encouraged to practise this as their own self-hypnosis routine to reduce anxiety before the feared procedure and to cope with pain and discomfort during it.

Using a related approach, one young client with needle phobia was able to tolerate a routine immunisation injection in front of her classmates by learning in hypnosis to experience her arm as becoming detached from her body and to then use the same strategy in the real situation – leaving her arm with the nurse while the injection took place. For dental phobics it is often helpful to teach a hypnotised client how to make their hand feel numb (by imagining plunging it into snow for example) and to transfer that numbness by touching an appropriate part of their mouth – which they can then do later when in the dental chair. With chronic pain, such as that associated with fibromyalgia, some clients are able to reduce their painful experience in hypnosis by 'turning down' an imaginary 'dial' that controls their pain. One person who was suffering from a disabling chronic pain that had continued long after a whiplash injury had physically healed found she could divert her pain in self-hypnosis to the top of her head, where it would be released 'like lava spurting out of a volcano'. Similarly, a client with phantom limb pain, which she described like a 'fizzling firework about to explode', was able to 'douse' the pain by imagining pouring a jug of water over it. Both of these clients went on to apply the same technique for themselves in everyday situations using a rapid self-hypnosis procedure and found that their pain throughout the day was significantly reduced and sometimes eliminated.

In addition to the treatment of fear of pain, hypnosis can also be used to reduce patients' experience of actual pain. Langenfeld (2000) tested the use of hypnosis in pain management for patients with AIDS. By the end of the 12-week period of the study, all patients reported experiencing less pain. Self-hypnosis has also been used effectively in pain control. Anbar (2001) found that four out of five children taught self-hypnotic techniques to help with recurrent, unexplained abdominal pain had ceased to experience pain within 3 weeks. Substantial pain relief can be achieved by direct hypnotic suggestion in 75% of the population and more complete analgesia in about 20% of hypnotic subjects (Montgomery *et al.* 2000) so, although it can be used with most people, it is not a solution available to all patients. For those individuals for whom it is effective, however, it is sufficient for analgesia during surgery, dentistry and to relieve persistent pain, such as in cancer or burns patients.

As might be expected, directly suggested analgesia is more effective in high-susceptibility subjects than those who are less susceptible (Montgomery *et al.* 2000). However, this relationship is not so evident when more broadly based hypnotic strategies are used. This suggests that some feature other than, or in addition to, direct suggestion is important in achieving the analgesia. These results may arise because low-susceptibility patients may be as good as high-susceptibility patients at employing more general pain-coping strategies explicitly offered by the hypnotist (such as relaxation and distraction). This view is supported by the observation that such strategies, including the use of suggestion, are often effective, without hypnosis, in producing analgesia (Spanos *et al.* 1974).

There is, however, experimental evidence demonstrating the occurrence of specific suggestion-based changes associated with the perception of pain under hypnosis. Rainville *et al.* (1997) used positron-emission tomography (PET) scanning to track brain changes during hypnosis and its effect on experimentally induced pain. They found that activity in a particular area of the brain, the anterior cingulate gyrus, remained unchanged when hypnosis was induced but did change in relation to suggestions about the unpleasantness of pain.

The process by which pain relief is mediated during hypnosis is unclear. Apart from the effects of relaxation and distraction, a possible explanation is that hypnosis activates the release of endorphins. If so, then naloxone should reverse the effects of hypnotically induced analgesia. However, the majority of studies that have looked at this have concluded that hypnotic analgesia is not dependent on endogenous opioid systems (Crawford and Gruzelier 1992) An alternative explanation for the mechanism by which hypnosis acts is that of belief in efficacy (Wadden and Anderton 1982). This suggests that hypnosis may be having a type of placebo effect but that this arises when it is perceived as a means to enable an existing procedure (such as therapy, surgery or drugs) to work. In these cases hypnosis may act to enhance the effectiveness of other treatment rather than to relieve pain or other symptoms itself.

This last possibility is consistent with the view that hypnosis is most effective when used alongside other techniques such as cognitive behavioural therapy (Kirsch *et al.* 1995). Oakley *et al.* (1996) observe that, in itself, hypnosis is not a form of therapy. Rather, it can be used as an adjunct – providing a context in which therapies can be delivered more effectively. Hence they reject the use of labels such as 'hypnotherapy'; being an effective therapist must be the starting point from which the additional deployment of hypnosis may be advantageous to clients.

Conclusions

Pain can be defined and, with variable reliability and validity, be measured in clinical settings and researched. The most commonly used tool for measuring pain is the McGill Pain Questionnaire, which assesses the intensity, location and emotional components of pain but does not differentiate well between different types of pain.

The gate control theory offers an effective explanation of pain that accounts for the roles of pain specific neurones, the spinal cord and a range of physical, emotional, behavioural and cognitive factors that can increase or decrease perception of pain. The exact mechanism by which such a gate could operate is still unclear, although evidence suggests a critical role for endorphins – natural opiate-like molecules. Endorphins appear also to be implicated in acupuncture and the placebo effect, although apparently not in hypnotic analgesia. Psychological variables of anxiety, conditioning, expectancy and cognitive dissonance all affect the perception of pain and they, too, relate to the placebo effect.

Patients' experience of pain depends on many factors, including their locus of control and deployment of emotion or problem-focused coping strategies. Physical interventions to reduce pain include analgesic medication, physical stimulation and surgery. Psychological strategies to enhance coping with pain including relaxation, biofeedback and hypnosis, have been shown to be effective for some patients and are becoming increasingly acceptable, in part because of the insight offered by the gate control theory.

Reflective activity

Imagine that you wake up one morning with a headache. Make a list of actions you could take that, according to the gate control theory, would make it better or worse. If you choose either to sit and think positively 'Maybe it will go soon' or to get up and fetch some paracetamol, are you behaving in an emotion-focused or problem-focused way? Think about the way you actually respond to having a headache. Does your behaviour reflect an internal locus of control, suggesting that you believe that you can do something about the pain, or an external locus, believing that the progress of the headache is beyond your control?

Rapid recap

Check your progress so far by working through each of the following questions.

1. Describe one way in which pain is measured in a clinical setting and one way in which it can be measured for the purposes of research.

2. Too much work on a computer or reading a book can lead to an eye-strain headache. How would the gate control theory of pain account for the effectiveness of rubbing one's eyes to relieve the pain?

3. Vinar (1969) reported a case study of an individual who had become dependent upon a placebo. Use the idea of expectation to explain how this situation might have arisen.

If you have difficulty with more than one of the questions, read through the section again to refresh your understanding before moving on.

Key references

Other references are in the main reference list at the end of the book.

De Craen, A.J.M., Roos, P.J., de Vries, A.L. and Kleijnen, J. (1996) Effect of colour of drugs: systematic review of perceived effect of drugs and of their effectiveness. *British Medical Journal*, **313**: 1624–1626.

Kirsch, I., Montgomery, G. and Sapirstein, G. (1995) Hypnosis as an adjunct to cognitve-behavioral therapy: a meta-analysis. *Journal of Consulting and Clinical Psychology*, **63**: 214–220.

Melzack, R. and Wall, P.D. (1965) Pain mechanisms: a new theory. *Science*, **150**: 971–979.

Oakley, D., Alden, P. and Degun Mather, M. (1996) The use of hypnosis in therapy with adults. *Psychologist*, **9**: 502–505.

Ogden, J. (2000) *Health Psychology: A textbook*. Open University Press, Buckingham.

Taylor, S.E. (1995) *Health Psychology*. McGraw-Hill, New York.

6

Bereavement and grief

I ndividuals differ in their experience and expression of **grief** and in the time they take to come to terms with the loss. In addition, differences in responses to **bereavement** may arise out of culturally determined patterns of behaviour following a death. Such differences must be respected, yet health care staff must be vigilant to detect individuals for whom grieving extends beyond the typical range of experience in terms of emotional extremes or time. This chapter considers first the generalisations that can be made about grieving and both common individual and social differences and unusual, pathological, patterns of grief. Nurses are exposed to more death than virtually any other profession so need to be prepared to offer help to the bereaved. Conversely, such constant contact with death can be stressful and health care professionals need support services too.

The process of bereavement

The health care service aims to promote, sustain and recover the health of patients. Although it is inevitable, it is nevertheless distressing when this process cannot succeed and a patient dies. As a consequence, health care staff, who may themselves be affected by the death, will be called upon to inform bereaved relatives and offer them support in their grief.

In addition to the suffering of grief, the bereaved may have other issues to deal with such as arranging a funeral and dealing with the dead person's personal effects. These are not of immediate consequence to health psychology, although, as a source of stress (Chapter 4), the death of a loved one has health implications in itself so such responsibilities can add to the burden, negatively affecting the health of the bereaved. Clearly, the importance of stress to the negative impact of bereavement is indicated by the greater debilitation experienced by those whose loved ones have died in traumatic circumstances rather than peacefully (Jacobs 1999).

Learning outcomes

By the end of this chapter you should be able to:

- Describe the stages through which a bereaved individual passes during the grieving process
- Understand differences in the grieving process between individuals, including social and cultural differences
- Identify ways in which bereaved individuals and health care staff can be supported when a patient dies.

⚷ Keywords

....

Grief
The emotional reaction to bereavement

Bereavement
The experience of the death of a person whom an individual knows closely

Bartrop *et al.* (1977), using non-bereaved controls, and Schleifer *et al.* (1983) who compared pre- and post-bereavement measures, found that bereaved individuals had impaired immune responses. This could be linked to stress (Chapter 4) and therefore account for the increased risk of illness experienced by people who have suffered a loss through death. Bereaved people are even at greater risk of dying themselves (Parkes *et al.* 1969, Siegel and Kuykendall 1990), especially if they are male (Bowling 1987). Of course, this could be explained in other ways, such as a loss of social support (see also Chapter 2) or by the simple consequences of being alone, such as having a greater workload or being unable to afford healthy foods. Gass (1989) reported that widows and widowers had greater tobacco, alcohol and tranquilliser use than non-bereaved controls. Widowers were particularly likely to drink to excess and this may account for the finding that cirrhosis of the liver is more prevalent in this group (Stroebe and Stroebe 1983).

Symptoms of grief

Physical symptoms

- Tightness in the throat
- Breathlessness and the need to sigh
- Feeling of hollowness or emptiness
- Bodily weakness and lack of energy
- Bodily aches and pains

Behavioural symptoms

- Loss of appetite
- Insomnia
- Repetitious behaviour
- Social withdrawal
- Carrying reminders of the deceased
- Searching for the deceased

Cognitive symptoms

- Denial
- Difficulty concentrating
- Memory problems
- Dreams of the deceased
- Hallucinations of the deceased

Emotional symptoms

- Numbness
- Sadness
- Anger
- Guilt
- Depression
- Yearning
- Loneliness
- Helplessness
- Relief

⊶ᴀ Keywords

Neurosis
A state of unrealistic anxiety

Sometimes grieving is unusually intense or entirely absent (when it would be expected); these are instances of pathological grief. The latter may result from **repression** of grief, which, it is assumed, can lead to later psychological symptoms such as **neurosis**. Although there is evidence to support the idea of repression in general

O—ℼ *Keywords*

Repression

A state in which access to traumatic memories is prevented. Freud suggests that they remain in the unconscious – in order to protect the individual's conscious awareness – but such memories can consequentially cause disturbances to mental health

O—ℼ *Keywords*

Mourning

The socially and culturally dictated ways of expressing grief

(e.g. Koehler *et al.* 2002), the relationship with pathological grief is only assumed. There is, in fact, evidence to the contrary. Wortman and Silver (1987) found that in their sample of parents of children who died in infancy, those who had 'worked through' their feelings, expressing their grief, showed greater and more prolonged distress at their loss. In chronic grief the sorrow associated with the loss lasts for many years and may arise as a consequence of the bereaved person having had an ambivalent relationship with the deceased that prevents them from accepting the death (Parkes 1975).

Delayed grief arises when the loss is ignored or denied but eventually accepted. This can occur if grieving is difficult, such as for a parent who loses a partner but tries to suppress his or her feelings in order to ease the pain of the loss experienced by their children. Absent grief may occur if a death is not confirmed, for example, if the body of a murder victim is not found. In either case, some later event, such as another loss, may trigger the delayed grieving process (Worden 1991).

Stages in the bereavement process

Grief follows bereavement but its exact pattern depends on the bereaved individual, the nature of the death and the characteristic **mourning** of the society. Some individuals experience little grief – for example, those people who feel that the death represents a relief from suffering for the dead person (although this is not always the case in such circumstances). For most bereaved people, the grieving process may last for weeks, months or even years. During the early stages, the bereaved can expect considerable social support, offering both emotional solace and practical help. However, when this ceases the grieving process is rarely over and the bereaved person may feel very lonely with neither their loved one nor the previous level of social support. This sense of abandonment and isolation is exemplified in the following passage: 'Grief following bereavement by death is aggravated if the person lost is the person to whom one would turn in times of trouble. Faced with the biggest trouble she has ever had, the widow repeatedly finds herself turning toward the person who is not there' (Parkes 2000, p. 327).

Two generalised descriptions of the grieving process have been suggested by Kübler-Ross (1969) and Parkes (1972) (see box on page 210). However, as people vary in their experience of the grief process, it has been argued that it is more useful to identify the tasks to be achieved through mourning. Worden (1991) suggested that these are:

- accepting the reality of the loss
- working through the pain

- adjusting to the absence of the deceased from the environment
- moving forward in life.

Even within this wider remit, individual differences will arise, with people taking differing lengths of time over some tasks or failing to achieve them at all.

Two models of grieving

Kübler-Ross (1969) proposed a five stage process of adjusting to death:

- Denial
- Anger
- Bargaining
- Depression
- Acceptance.

Parkes (1972) identified four phases of mourning:

- Numbness
- Yearning and denial
- Disorganisation and despair
- Reorganisation.

Initially, a bereaved person is likely to experience pain, numbness or desolation. Through this 'haze' they may deny that the loss is real or permanent. Such feelings are common and often intense; the bereaved person may feel unable to think or do anything and cannot contemplate ever feeling differently. Health care professionals need to be aware that this apparent detachment from reality is common and does not represent a genuine failure to accept that their loved one is dead.

Simultaneously, or subsequently, the bereaved individual may experience strong feelings of guilt and/or anger. They may blame themselves for the death, or resent the dead person for leaving them and later they may 'bargain', trying to find ways to reverse the loss. Again, this stage has the potential to present health care staff with problems as they may feel drawn into the bereaved person's essentially private crisis.

During these early stages of grief, an important marker may be a leave-taking ceremony, such as a funeral. This allows the bereaved to make a statement of farewell to the deceased. There are gender differences in this respect, with women benefiting from the funeral as this may represent a transition for them to a more senior role in the family or may boost their confidence as they successfully organise the event and are acknowledged for doing so. For men, however, a funeral may represent a hurdle rather than a comfort, particularly as they may feel that displaying emotion is inappropriate but may not be confident that they can fulfil this social convention. Following the funeral, the bereaved person may also experience greater loneliness as social support reduces. This may be exacerbated by the need to demonstrate social withdrawal as a mark of respect.

Depression and despair are commonly believed to be inevitable reactions to the death of someone close and although crying and intense sadness are common it is not the case that there is an absolute absence of positive emotions. Wortman and Silver (1987) (see also page 209) found that bereaved parents experienced intense emotions, including slightly more happiness than sadness, throughout the grieving period. Women more than men may find that they need to continuously replay events surrounding the death. In this process, called obsessional review, the loved one is recalled in a positive light, allowing the bereaved individual to feel positive emotions. This may provide a way to come to terms with the death.

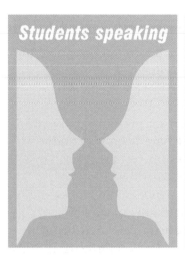

Students speaking

A first experience of a patient dying . . .

A final year nursing student

I remember the nurse I was working with when I had to care for a patient who had died for the first time in my career. She suggested that I talk to the deceased person as I might normally, but I felt a bit uncomfortable about this. I do feel that this is a really important job, doing the last thing for them in as peaceful way as possible. I find it is much harder if I have known the patient for a long time, as it is more upsetting when you have to lay this person out.

The final stage is reorganisation: as the bereaved individual starts to cope they restructure their life in the absence of their loved one. Even in cases where the death has been anticipated this may take many months, partly because cultural norms dictate that it is 'improper' to prepare for a death. In relationships where each person played a distinct role, this task may require that the bereaved individual learns a new set of skills such as household management or car maintenance. The establishment of a new relationship may be difficult to consider for the bereaved person or for others to accept.

Reflective activity

If you have experienced the death of a patient on a placement, can you identify any of these stages in the relatives, other patients on the ward or staff?

Individual differences in grieving

Gender differences

Women tend to display more overt grief than men (Glick *et al.* 1974) and are more likely to suffer obsessional grief. However, they are also more likely to benefit from attending a funeral (page 210) and are less likely to turn to alcohol than men. There are also gender differences in the way that bereavement is experienced. Women describe feelings of abandonment whereas men describe feeling dismembered. For heterosexual couples this can be understood in terms of the meaning of marriage for women – as a key social relationship. So, for a widow, returning to work may help to satisfy the loss of her interpersonal relationship. Emotional responses also differ between widows and widowers: women tend to feel angry and cry, wanting someone to sort their life out for them, whereas men feel 'choked up' and guilty. Although they are better at accepting the death of their partner in some respects, making a faster social recovery, widowers take longer to overcome the emotional consequences.

For homosexual couples, loss of the partner presents additional difficulties. Although the relationship may have been long and committed, the remaining individual is not (as yet) recognised by the state as next of kin. The grieving survivor will be just as emotionally distressed as a heterosexual partner would be, yet they may not be accepted or even known to the family so may be excluded from activities that form an important part of the grieving process (such as the funeral or post-mortem, if there is one). Health care professionals need to be aware of this risk.

In the past, despite positive beliefs, health care staff may have unwittingly demonstrated homophobic behaviour. Smith (1993) found that, although the majority of nurses tested showed neutral or slightly positive attitudes towards gays and lesbians, they also indicated predominantly moderate (57%) or severe (20%) homophobia. So, whilst health care staff may have expressed positive views about gay people, this was not necessarily reflected in their feelings towards their patients. More recent evidence, however, presents a more optimistic picture, with Erlen *et al.* (1999) finding a very low incidence of homophobic attitudes among nurses (an average score of 1.14 on a range of 0–28). Gay couples may, however, be advantaged in one respect in relation to heterosexuals. McDougall (1993) reviewed the literature on ageing in homosexual men and women and found that, because gay relationships are flexible in the roles that each individual takes, when death occurs the bereaved individual may cope better.

Adjusting to traumatic deaths

Grieving is less pronounced following the death of an elderly compared to a younger person (Ball 1977). This difference may arise because of the unexpected nature of death in the young. Where death is due to an accident or suicide, however, grief is more intense (Shanfield *et al.* 1987, Range and Calhoun 1990).

Dyregrov *et al.* 2003

Aim: To investigate differences in distress experienced by parents whose young children die through suicide, sudden infant death syndrome (SIDS) or accident.

Procedure: The distress experienced by 232 parents from 140 families bereaved by traumatic death (suicide, SIDS or accident) was investigated $1\frac{1}{2}$ years after the loss.

Findings: More than half of the participants were still suffering grief reactions. There were no significant differences between parents of children who had lost a child through suicide or through accident, although both showed greater distress than parents bereaved by SIDS. The best predictor of distress was social isolation.

Conclusion: Sudden and traumatic deaths of children have lasting effects on grieving parents, especially if they receive less social support.

Faulkner (1995) identifies several circumstances in which bereavement is particularly difficult to adjust to:

● Violent death, e.g. murder
● If the deceased and bereaved had a difficult relationship, either high-dependence or strongly negative
● If the bereaved has suffered multiple losses (through other deaths, divorce or mutilating surgery).

In these situations, both men and women experience more difficulties in coming to terms with their loss.

Effects of death on others who are ill

There are some situations in which people may be more likely to know others who are terminally ill, for example among sufferers with acquired immune deficiency syndrome (AIDS). In the early years of the disease some social groups, such as gay men, had high incidence rates for AIDS. This had two consequences: a greater stigmatisation of those who were human immunodeficiency virus (HIV)-positive or perceived to be at risk, and exposure of individuals to multiple deaths of their peers at a relatively young age. Since anticipation of someone's death can exacerbate grief, and because bereavement is emotionally taxing, multiply bereaved individuals may suffer significantly more distress (Martin 1988). The pattern of such grieving, however, is predictable, characterised by crying, preoccupation with the deceased and feelings of yearning and denial. The same factors are important in improving coping. For example, adequate social support, or at least the perception of having sufficient support if it were needed, appears to help bereaved gay men to cope with their loss (Lennon *et al.* 1990).

There are several sources of stress relating to HIV and AIDS: the effect of bereavement, the risk of infection (or of progression of the disease for those who are HIV-positive) and the stigmatisation associated with the disease. For gay men a further source of associated stress is homophobia. Sodroski *et al.* (1984) suggest that such distress may increase the replication rate of the virus, accelerating the onset of AIDS. Reed *et al.* (1999) found that HIV-positive men who had experienced the loss of a close friend or partner were more likely to show signs of disease progression (as indicated by **CD4 T-helper** cell levels). However, this pattern was not consistent. Men who maintained their CD4 T-helper cell levels were more likely to have managed to find purpose in their loss. For example, if the bereaved individual had been prompted into action to enjoy the time they had left they were less likely to demonstrate a decline. This finding is in line with the predictions of Taylor's cognitive adaptation model (1983), which suggests that searching for meaning and ultimately feeling empowered by mastery over a threatening event allows an individual to cope.

⌐ₙ Keywords
....

CD4 T-helper cell
A type of cell produced by the immune system. Fewer of these cells are found in patients with rapidly progressing HIV infection

media watch   **It's true: a healthy mind can cure**

It's what New Age healers have known all along: the mind does matter.

A study has shown that a positive state of mind can be almost as effective as drugs at fighting serious disease.

Researchers found that therapy can significantly reduce the amount of HIV virus in gay men suffering from the disease. It is the first to show that counselling can have such a dramatic impact.

'From now on every single doctor treating HIV – and many other serious diseases – should think hard about helping patients with their mental health, so

continued

the outcome of the treatment will be better. It's not enough just to give people pills,' said Dr Alberto Avendaño, director of HIV services at the University of Maryland's Department of Family Medicine.

Earlier research has suggested a link between grief and a weakened immune system. Doctors also know that stress can exacerbate many illnesses.

However, the study, published in the *Journal of Human Virology*, is the first to show how actively giving therapy to people can lead to an immediate improvement in their physical health.

More than 100 gay men who were HIV-positive and had lost a partner from AIDS in the previous six months were split into two groups. One set was given grief therapy and the other sent on a community programme. The therapy encouraged crying and venting, figuring out how to face the future, and learning ways to deal with stress.

Blood tests were given before and after the 10 sessions, and it was found that the therapy significantly reduced the amount of the HIV virus in men. The changes reflected a marked improvement in the patients' physical wellbeing.

Anthony Browne, Health Editor *The Observer*, Sunday 4 March 2001, page 11

Over to you

From the evidence you have encountered so far, try to explain why counselling might affect the immune system and replication of the virus in relation to coping with grief.

Keywords

Anticipatory grieving

Emotions experienced because of a predicted loss, such as when a patient has a terminal illness. Although it can help an individual to prepare for the impending death, the prolonged process of separation can worsen emotional coping

Anticipatory grieving

Pearlin *et al.* (1989) describe the feelings of **anticipatory grieving** experienced by people who care for Alzheimer's sufferers. They identify feelings of loss resembling bereavement while the individual is still alive because the person they once knew no longer exists. Such caregivers may experience emotions including anger, fear of abandonment as the relationship deteriorates, depression and sleeplessness (Soukup 1996). Physiological changes in anticipatory grief, including immunosuppression, have also be identified (Kiecolt-Glaser *et al.* 1987). In addition, Kiecolt-Glaser *et al.* (1988) found that if carers themselves have good social support, they tend to cope better. However, if illness is prolonged (beyond 6 months), grief may be worsened (Gerber *et al.* 1975). Clukey (2003) interviewed carers experiencing anticipatory grieving in relation to a family member. She described additional emotions, including sadness, feeling overwhelmed or trapped, frustration and guilt. These closely reflect the experiences of grief after a death.

Cultural differences in grieving

Many societies have clear cultural rituals for responding to bereavement. Whilst some of these may be more positive than others – celebrating the dead person's life rather than mourning their death – a socially determined pattern of responses could help to make grieving easier. The presence of social guidelines for the bereaved and those with whom they come into contact reduces stress. Walter *et al.* (2000) suggest that, in Britain, traditionally explicit expectations about the behaviour of grieving people do not exist; no longer are widows expected to dress in black and wear a veil nor widowers to wear a black armband.

In some cultures, however, such conventions guide the expression of grief in the bereaved. The Irish wake, which may include a feast, allows the body to be watched by relatives for several days until the burial. In contrast, the customs surrounding bereavement for orthodox Jews determine when the bereaved leave the house, how they dress and when recreation can be enjoyed. Exactly one year after the death, mourning is completed by the dedication of the tombstone. Traditional Japanese death rituals aim to enable the deceased to travel to a better place. Loved ones assist this journey with ceremonies, ritual bathing of the corpse and a feast that returns the mourners to the community. The Hindu religion views life and death as a cycle; thus death is a transitional state before rebirth.

The absence of tradition and 'stiff upper lip' attitude prevalent in Britain (and in America), in which the role of the bereaved in dealing with the practicalities of the death is much reduced, may not, ultimately, benefit everyone trying to come to terms with a loss. So, when health care professionals encounter bereaved individuals they must consider their cultural as well as individual needs in terms of expressing their grief.

Children's experience of bereavement

As adults, we expect, ultimately, that we will experience bereavement, but bereavement during childhood is also surprising common. One in 30 children will have experienced the death of a parent by the time they are 19 and their response to this experience is different from that of adults. Children suffer many of the same emotions, of guilt, anger, numbness and depression, but their response is less predictable than that of adults.

Another important difference between children and adults is the child's differing understanding of the concept of death. Nagy (1948) described three developmental stages in a child's comprehension of the meaning of death:

- **Age 3–5 years** – death as separation or a diminished form of life, a reversible state like sleeping
- **Age 5/6–9 years** – death as final, a permanent state but one that can be evaded and is neither universal nor personal
- **Age 10** – death as universal and inevitable, including the child's own eventual death.

Age affects understanding of death

Although the exact ages will vary with individual children, the general pattern of progressive understanding has been supported by subsequent research. It is important for health carers who are working with bereaved children to recognise that they will have a concept of death and may need, as much as adults, to express and discuss their thoughts and feelings (Brookes 2002).

Davis (1989) observed that children are often misinformed or uninformed about death and, as a consequence, are denied the right to grieve. Through art therapy, Davis suggests, children can be given permission to express their emotions without fear of disapproval. Using puppets, drawing, story telling and clay modelling, art therapy allows children to become aware of and display their feelings, work them through and enjoy the experience.

Helping bereaved individuals

Support for families

Imparting bad news is difficult; because it is hard to receive news of death, it is therefore hard to give. It is advisable to avoid sidestepping the issue, beginning with as little introductory information possible, perhaps just identifying health care staff present and their roles, then providing information about the death as gently as possible without disguising it – the message must be honest and open. Communication needs to be clear and consistent, the use of expressions such as 'expired' or 'no longer with us' are not helpful, they simple have the potential to lead to confusion.

Once individuals have learned of their loss they need support. Health care staff have a key role here. It is advisable to:

- Listen to what is said
- Stay calm
- Accept the emotions that are displayed (such as anger or an absence of response in a silent recipient)
- Give the bereaved person time to process the information given to them
- Accept and not disguise your own sadness, without burdening them further.

It is also inadvisable to:

- Attempt to explain how you feel or you previous experiences
- Attempt to justify why this has happened.

Once the bereaved person has said all they want to, further assistance is important. Following a death, bereaved individuals are likely to be shocked and may find new tasks difficult. Health care staff can provide initial information and reassurance that many bereaved individuals will need about what will happen next. Such information will include:

- The need for a relative to take a copy of the death certificate issued by the doctor certifying the death to the Registrar of Births, Marriages and Deaths
- Possibly the need for a post-mortem examination and, if so, the potential for delay in issuing a death certificate
- How to find an undertaker (without making specific recommendations).

Reassurance at this stage may include the need to:

- Talk through a request for a post-mortem
- Allay fears about mutilation of the dead person's body
- Accept that undertakers can help the family with many organisational aspects of dealing with the death, not just organising the funeral.

Community District
Nurse

Professionally speaking . . .

Caring for dying patients

We can be involved with a family for weeks/months/years before somebody dies and during that time we've built up a relationship not just with the patient but with the husband, or wife, the children and the neighbours. We all put terminal patients at the top of the list. It's all part of case-load management and you get better at that by doing it.

I do all the initial assessments, and anything where the other staff are unsure. I get involved with the more complex cases, early stages of palliative care. People want to have one person going in that they have to relate to. It's not helpful to have various nurses popping in because they have to go over and over the same things. Probably a lot of the early palliative care I will do that for as it requires quite expert practice and as the physical care needs increase I will introduce the other team members.

It can be very tough, we had a really bad patch, we'd been busy all year with palliative care, and we had about four patients all very ill at the same time. That was very tough because we were trying to keep the patients symptom-free, and dealing with the grief is very time-consuming. That's when being part of an extended team is a help because we do try and help each other out. We all know about the terminal patients because we all cover them at the weekends. We give each other a lot of support.

I think you need to ensure a mix of clients. Not spending your whole time with patients who are dying. However, there is a satisfaction when it goes right. A peaceful home death, and everyone has done what they wanted to do. With one client it went like a dream and it was indescribably satisfying, and the letter from the family made me cry they were so appreciative.

In addition, health care staff can observe reactions of bereaved individuals and in cases of concern it may be appropriate to alert community nurses. Macmillan nurses, for example, visit bereaved relatives as a matter of course. Keeping in contact with relatives after the death is important as they may harbour feelings or beliefs about the patient's life or illness that they cannot come to terms with. Nurses may find that they are asked to help, for example taking away equipment or medicines that act as reminders of the loss. This can provide an opportunity to allow bereaved individuals to talk about their emotions or about their loved one.

Over to you

Find out about the provision for bereaved people in your local area. Is bereavement counselling offered at your local hospitals or Macmillan hospice if you have one? Look at the advertisements in Yellow Pages for Funeral Services offered in your area. What range of services is provided? Do you have a local branch of Cruse? Does your own doctors' surgery have information about funeral directors? Finally, consider how aware someone might be of any of these services in the event of an unexpected death – how much of what you discovered was new to you?

Health care staff will have priorities of their own, such as removing personal belongings from the hospital, and these needs should be expressed with due consideration for the feelings of the bereaved individuals.

In the longer term, a range of services is available to people who have suffered bereavement and for those enduring anticipatory grieving. These include:

- Individual counselling
- Group therapy
- Family therapy with the dying person in a hospice setting
- Support groups of similarly affected individuals.

Evidence suggests that such support is beneficial as it reduces the risk of subsequent psychological disorders (Parkes 1980). One way in which these services may be of use is in allowing the bereaved individual to 'work through' their grief, as suggested by Worden (1991; see page 209). However, not all people desire such assistance and, as Zisook *et al.* (1995) observe, there is little reliable evidence about the efficacy of different kinds of provision because success of services is not measured in a consistent way.

Other aspects of adjustment are the need to replace lost social support and to regain control. Many bereaved people throw themselves into work or new relationships following the loss of a loved one. By so doing, they may achieve replacement control or social support. Bereavement counselling should enable individuals to seek a workable balance between these needs. In the short term, counselling itself provides social support and encourages the individual to take control of their own existence, a strategy that will, in turn, lead to sources of social support.

Support for staff

Apart from servicemen and -women in wartime, nursing staff are exposed to death more often than people in any other profession. Unsurprisingly, this can at times be traumatic. Valente (2003) found that health care professionals were significantly affected by a patient's death by suicide, experiencing feelings of guilt and responsibility, and Tyler *et al.* (1991) found that, for nurses in both private and public health services, high workload and the need to cope with death and dying were the most frequently cited causes of stressful experiences at work. Similarly, DesCamp *et al.* (1993) found exposure to death and dying to be among the three most important stressors for nursing staff. Although they anticipated that humour at work would help to buffer the effects of stress, it did not do so significantly. The use of high levels of active, physical play did counteract job and workload stress, however. Davis (1989), who has recommended the use of art therapy with bereaved children, suggests that this strategy could also offer an outlet for stressed health care staff. Many of the same facilities available to families can be of benefit to staff. Social support and counselling are important factors in enabling health care workers to cope with their job stressors. Counselling services for nurses are offered by the Royal College of Nursing and all NHS Trusts are required to provide counselling facilities for their staff.

Conclusions

Bereavement almost always leads to grief, although the extent of grieving is variable. In general, feelings such as numbness and denial are followed by anger, despair and depression. Initially, bereaved individuals feel as though they cannot cope but, over time, most come to terms with their loss and reorganise their lives. Grief may result in a range of physical, behavioural, cognitive and emotional responses. For some individuals, the cultural demands of mourning, such as the funeral, are helpful, although this differs, for instance between men and women. Other differences in grieving arise as a result of the nature of the death (for example whether it was traumatic or was expected) and whether the individual has suffered many losses.

A grieving response can also occur in advance of death, for example in carers looking after patients with Alzheimer's disease. This anticipatory grieving can be very prolonged and distressing but does not necessarily prepare the grieving individual for the death when it does come.

Children's understanding of death develops slowly. Nevertheless, they are entitled to the opportunity to grieve.

Health care staff are regularly faced with trying to assist bereaved individuals. Being initially calm and accepting allows bereaved individuals the opportunity to express their immediate feelings if they wish. Subsequently, being prepared to continue to listen and offering practical advice and reassurance are key roles. Eventually, formal services may be offered to bereaved individuals to help them to cope. The vigilance of health care staff to potential problems is important at this stage.

Finally, health care staff themselves may experience grief at the loss of patients and resources to assist in coping with the stresses of professional life are available.

Over to you

Imagine a child who is in hospital awaiting treatment, whose parent is killed. They haven't said 'goodbye' and cannot attend the funeral. What emotions are they likely to experience and what assistance might they need? How would their grief differ if they were 4 or 7 years old?

RRRRRRapid recap

Check your progress so far by working through each of the following questions.

1. How does the idea proposed by Worden (1991) differ from the stage processes described by Kübler-Ross and Parkes and why might Worden's approach be more useful?

2. a. Identify four differences between the grieving of men and women.

   b. Will all men and women differ in these ways?

   c. In what ways is the experience of bereaved children similar to and different from that of adults?.

3. The problem pages of magazines often describe the misery of people who care for a relative with a progressive disease, such as multiple sclerosis, who feel as though they are grieving before their relative has even died. How would you explain what they were experiencing if you were asked to do so by a hospital visitor expressing similar concerns?

If you have difficulty with more than one of the questions, read through the section again to refresh your understanding before moving on.

Key references

Other references are in the main reference list at the end of the book.

Bartrop, R.W., Luckhurst, E., Lazarus, L. *et al.* (1977) Depressed lymphocyte function after bereavement. *Lancet*, **1**, 834–836.

Davis, C.B. (1989) The use of art therapy and group process with grieving children. *Issues in Comprehensive Pediatric Nursing*, **12**: 269–280.

DesCamp, K.D. and Thomas, C.C. (1993) Buffering nursing stress through play at work. *Western Journal of Nursing Research*, **15**: 619–627.

Gerber, L., Rusalem, R. and Hannon, N. (1975) Anticipatory grief and aged widows and widowers. *Journal of Gerontology*, **30**: 225–229.

Parkes, C.M., Benjamin, B. and Fitzgerald, R.G. (1969) Broken heart: a statistical study of increased mortality among widowers. *British Medical Journal*, **1**: 740–743.

Smith, G.B. (1993) Homophobia and attitudes toward gay men and lesbians by psychiatric nurses. *Archives of Psychiatric Nursing*, **7**: 377–384.

References

Abraham, C. and Sheeran, P. (1993) In search of a psychology of safer-sex promotion: beyond beliefs and text. *Health Education Research: Theory and Practice*, **8**: 245–254.

Abraham, C. and Sheeran, P. (1994) Modelling and modifying young heterosexuals' HIV-preventative behaviour: a review of theories, findings and educational implications. *Patient Education and Counseling*, **23**: 173–186.

Abraham, C., Sheeran, P., Spears, R. and Abrams, D. (1992) Health beliefs and the promotion of HIV-preventative infections among teenagers: a Scottish perspective. *Health Psychology*, **11**: 363–370.

Abram, H.S., Moore, G.L. and Westervelt, F.B. (1971) Suicidal behavior in chronic dialysis patients. *American Journal of Psychiatry*, **127**: 1199–1204.

Acton, W.I. (1970) Speech intelligibility in a background noise and noise-induced hearing loss. *Ergonomics*, **13**: 546–554.

Affleck, G., Urrows, S., Tennen, H. and Higgins, P. (1992) Daily coping with pain from rheumatoid arthritis: patterns and correlates. *Pain*, **51**: 221–229.

Ajzen, I. (1985) From intentions to actions: a theory of planned behavior. In: *Action-control: From cognition to behavior* (eds J. Kuhl and J. Beckman). Springer, Heidelberg, pp. 11–39.

Ajzen, I. (1991) The theory of planned behavior. *Organizational Behavior and Human Decision Processes*, **50**: 179–211.

Ajzen, I. and Fishbein, M. (1980) *Understanding attitudes and predicting social behavior*. Prentice-Hall, Englewood Cliffs, NJ.

Anbar, R.D. (2001) Self-hypnosis for the treatment of functional abdominal pain in childhood. *Clinical Pediatrics*, **40**: 447–451.

Anderson, J.L., Dodman, S., Kopelman, M. and Fleming, A. (1979) Patient information recall in a rheumatology clinic. *Rheumatology and Rehabilitation*, **18**: 18–22.

Andrews, A. and Carroll, M. (1998) Bilinguals' memory for medical information: effects of modality, type of information and order of information. *Psychology and Health*, **13**: 443–449.

Armstrong, D., Glanville, T., Bailey, E. and O'Keefe, G. (1990) Doctor-initiated consultations: a study of communication between general practitioners and patients about the need for reattendance. *British Journal of General Practice*, **40**: 241–242.

Atkinson, R.C. and Shiffrin, R.M. (1968) Human memory: a proposed system and its control processes. In: *The Psychology of Learning and Motivation*, vol. 2 (eds K.W. Spence and J.T. Spence). London, Academic Press.

Ausburn, L. (1981) Patient compliance with medication regimes. In: *Advances in Behavioural Medicine*, vol. 1 (ed. J.L. Shepherd). Sydney, Cumberland College.

Bachman, J.G., Johnson, L.D., O'Malley, P.M. and Humphreys, H. (1988) Explaining the recent decline in marijuana use: differentiating the effects of perceived risk, disapproval, and general life-style factors. *Journal of Health and Social Behaviour*, **29**: 92–112.

Bales, R.F. (1970) *Personality and Interpersonal Behaviour*. Holt, Rinehart & Winston, New York.

Ball, J.F. (1977) Widow's grief: the impact of age and mode of death. *Omega*, **7**: 307–333.

Banbury, S. and Berry, D.C. (1998) Disruption of office-related tasks by speech and office noise. *British Journal of Psychology*, **89**: 499–517.

Bandura, A. (1992) Exercise of personal agency through the self-efficacy mechanism. In: *Self-Efficacy: Thought control and action* (ed. R. Schwarzer). Hemisphere, Washington, DC.

Baron, R.M., Mandel, D.R., Adams, C.A. and Griffen, L.M. (1976) Effects of social density in university residential environments. *Journal of Personality and Social Psychology*, **34**: 434–446.

Barrera, M. Jr, Sandler, I.N. and Ramsey, T.B. (1981) Preliminary development of a scale of social support: studies on college students. *American Journal of Community Psychology*, **9**: 435–447.

Bartrop, R.W., Luckhurst, E., Lazarus, L. *et al.* (1977) Depressed lymphocyte function after bereavement. *Lancet*, **1**: 834–836.

Basbaum, A.I. and Fields, H.L. (1984) Endogenous pain control systems: brainstem spinal pathways and endorphin circuitry. *Annual Review of Neuroscience*, **7**: 309–338.

Basler, H.D. and Rehfisch, H.P. (1990) Follow up results of a cognitive behavioural treatment for chronic pain in a primary care setting. *Psychology and Health*, **4**: 293–304.

Baum, A. and Valins, S. (1977) *Architecture and social behavior: Psychological studies of social density*. Lawrence Erlbaum, Hillsdale, NJ.

Becker, M.H. (1979) Understanding patient compliance: the contributions of attitudes and other psychosocial factors. In: *New Directions in Patient Compliance* (ed. S.J. Cohen). Lexington Books, Lexington, MA.

Becker, M.H. and Maiman, L.A. (1980) Strategies for enhancing patient compliance. *Journal of Community Health*, **6**: 113–135.

Beckman, H.B. and Frankel, R.M. (1984) The effect of physician behaviour on the collection of data. *Annals of International Medicine*, **101**: 692–696.

Beckman, H.B., Kaplan, S.H. and Frankel, R.M. (1989) Outcome based research on doctor-patient communication: a review. In: *Communicating with Medical Patients* (eds M. Stewart and D. Roter). Sage, Newbury Park, CA.

Beecher, H.K. (1956) Relationship of significance of wound to pain experience. *Journal of the American Medical Association*, **161**: 1609–1613.

Beecher, H.K. (1959) *Measurement of Subjective Responses*. Oxford University Press, New York.

Belloc, N.B. and Breslow, L. (1972) Relationship of physical health status and health practices. *Preventative Medicine*, **1**: 409–421.

Ben-Eliyahu, S., Yirmiya, R., Liebeskind, J.C. *et al.* (1991) Stress increases metastatic spread of mammary tumor in rats: evidence for mediation by the immune system. *Brain, Behavior and Immunity*, **5**: 193–205.

Berg, A.O. (1977) Placebos: a brief review for family physicians. *Journal of Family Practice*, **5**: 97–100.

Berkman, L.F. and Syme, S.L. (1979) Social networks, host resistance, and mortality: a nine-year follow-up of Almeda County residents. *American Journal of Epidemiology*, **109**: 186–204.

Bernstein, B. (1961) Social class and linguistic development: a theory of social learning. In: *Education, Economy and Society* (eds A.H. Halsey, J. Floyd and C.A. Anderson). Collier-Macmillan, London.

Bernstein Hyman, R., Baker, S., Ephrain, R. *et al.* (1994) Health Belief Model variables as predictors of screening mammography utilization. *Journal of Behavioural Medicine*, **17**: 391–406.

Berry, D.L., Wilkie, D.J., Thomas, C.R Jr and Fortner, P. (2003) Clinicians communicating with patients experiencing cancer pain. *Cancer Investigation*, **21**: 364–381.

Bertakis, K.D. (1977) The communication of information from physician to patient: a method for increasing retention and satisfaction. *Journal of Family Practice*, **5**: 217–222.

Bibace, R. and Walsh, M.E. (1979) Developmental stages in children's conceptions of illness. In: *Health Psychology – A Handbook* (eds G.C. Stone, F. Cohen and N.E. Alder). Jossey-Bass, San Francisco, CA.

Bishop, G.D. (1994) *Health Psychology: Integrating mind and body*. Allyn & Bacon, London.

Blackwell, B. (1997) From compliance to adherence: a quarter of a century of research. In: *Treatment Compliance and the Therapeutic Alliance* (ed. B. Blackwell). Harwood Academic Publishers, Amsterdam.

Blair, A. (1993) Social class and the contextualisation of illness experience. In: *Worlds of Illness: Biographical and cultural perspectives on health and disease* (ed. A. Radley). Routledge, London.

Blakey, V. and Frankland, J. (1995) Evaluating HIV prevention for women prostitutes in Cardiff. *Health Education Journal*, **54**: 131–142.

Blanchard, E.B., Martin, J.E. and Dubbert, P.M. (1988) *Non-drug Treatments for Essential Hypertension*. Pergamon Press, Elmsford, NY.

Blaxter, M. and Paterson, E. (1982) *Mothers and Daughters: A three generational study of health attitudes and behaviour.* Heinemann, London.

Bleda, P. and Bleda, E. (1978) Effects of sex and smoking on reactions to spatial invasion at a shopping mall. *Journal of Social Psychology*, **104**: 311–312.

Bluebond-Langner, M. (1977) Meanings of death to children. In: *New Meanings of Death* (ed. H. Feidel). McGraw-Hill, New York, pp. 47–66.

Borland, R. and Naccarella, L. (1991) Reactions to the 1989 *Quit Campaign: Results from the two telephone surveys*. Quit Evaluation Studies No. 5. Victorian Smoking and Health Program, Melbourne, Victoria.

Borrelli, B. and Mermelstein, R. (1994) Goal setting and behavior change in a smoking cessation program. *Cognitive Therapy and Research*, **18**: 69–82.

Borrill, C.S., Wall, T.D., West, M.A. *et al.* (1998) *Stress among NHS Staff: final report*. Institute of Work Psychology, University of Sheffield, Sheffield.

Botvin, G.J., Eng, A. and Williams, C.L. (1980) Preventing the onset of cigarette smoking through life skills training. *Preventative Medicine*, **9**: 135–143.

Bouchard, C., Temblay, A., Depres, J.P. *et al.* (1990) The response to long-term overfeeding in identical twins. *New England Journal of Medicine*, **322**: 1477–1487.

Bovbjerg, V.E., McCann, B.S., Brief, D.J. *et al.* (1995) Spouse support and long-term adherence to lipid-lowering diets. *American Journal of Epidemiology*, **141**: 451–460.

Bowling, A. (1987) The hospitalisation of death: should more people die at home? *Journal of Moral Ethics*, **9**: 158–161.

Bradshaw, P.W., Ley, P., Kincey, J.A. and Bradshaw, J. (1975) Recall of medical advice: comprehensibility and specificity. *British Journal of Social and Clinical Psychology*, **14**: 55–62.

Bragg, B.W. (1973) *Seat Belts – Good Idea, But Are They Too Much Bother? An analysis of the relationship between attitudes toward seat belts and reported seat belt use*. Department of Transport, Road and Motor Vehicle Traffic Safety, Ottawa.

Breslow, L. and Enstrom, J. (1980) Persistence of medical conditions, habits and their relation to mortality. *Preventive Medicine*, **9**: 469–483.

Breznitz, S. (1984) *Cry Wolf: The psychology of false alarms*. Lawrence Erlbaum Associates, Hillsdale, NJ.

Brookes, M. (2002) Bereavement. *Times Educational Supplement*, **13 September**: 15–18.

Broome, A. and Llewelyn, S. (1995) *Health Psychology: Processes and applications*. Chapman & Hall, London.

Brosky, M.E., Keefer, O.A., Hodges, J.S. *et al.* (2003) Patient perceptions of professionalism in dentistry. *Journal of Dental Education*, **67**: 909–915.

Brown, P.E. (1972) Use of acupuncture in major surgery. *Lancet*, **1**: 1328–1330.

Brown, S.C. and Park, D.C. (2002) Roles of age and familiarity in learning health information. *Educational Gerontology*, **28**: 695–710.

Brownell, K.D. and Wadden, T.A. (1992) Etiology and treatment of obesity: Understanding a serious, prevalent and refractory disorder. *Journal of Consulting and Clinical Psychology*, **60**: 505–517.

Brubaker, C. and Wickersham, D. (1990) Encouraging the practice of testicular self examination: a field application of the theory of reasoned action. *Health Psychology*, **9**: 154–163.

Bulpitt, C.J., Beevers,D.G., Butler, A. *et al.* (1989) The effects of anti-hypertensive drugs on sexual function in men and women: a report from the DHSS Hypertension Care Computing Project (DHCCP), *Journal of Human Hypertension*, **3**: 53–56.

Burton, A.K., Tillotson, K.M., Main, C.J. and Hollis, S. (1995) Psychosocial predictors of outcome in acute and sub-chronic low-back trouble. *Spine*, **20**: 722–728.

Bush, P.J. and Osterweis, M. (1978) Pathways to medicine use. *Journal of Health and Social Behavior*, **19**: 179–189.

Cahill, G.F. Jr, Etzwiler, D.D. and Freinkel, N. (1976) 'Control' and diabetes. *New England Journal of Medicine*, **294**: 1004–1005.

Calhoun, J.B. (1962) Population density and social pathology. *Scientific American*, **206**: 139–148.

Carney, R.M., Schechter, K. and Davis, T. (1983) Improving adherence to blood glucose testing in insulin-dependent diabetic children. *Behavior Therapy*, **14**: 247–254.

Carney, R.M., Freeland, K.E., Eisen, S.A., Rich, M.W. and Jaffe, A.S. (1995) Major depression and medical adherence in elderly patients with coronary artery disease. *Health Psychology*, **14**: 88–90.

Carter, A.J. and West, M.A. (1999) Sharing the load: teamwork in health care settings. In: *Stress in Health Care Professionals* (eds R.L. Payne and J. Frith-Cozens). John Wiley, Chichester: pp. 191–120.

Centre for Behavioural Research in Cancer (1992) *Health Warnings and Contents Labelling on Tobacco Products*. Centre for Behavioural Research in Cancer, Melbourne.

Chaiken, S. (1979) Communicator physical attractiveness and persuasion. *Journal of Personality and Social Psychology*, **37**, 1387–1497.

Chaiken, S. and Eagly, A.H. (1976) Communication modality as a determinant of message persuasiveness and message comprehensibility. *Journal of Personality and Social Psychology*, **34**, 605–614.

Chaitchik, S., Kreitler, S., Shaked, S. *et al.* (1992) Doctor–patient communication in a cancer ward. *Journal of Cancer Education*, **7**: 41–54.

Chao, D.M., Shen, L.L., Tjen-A-Looi, S. *et al.* (1999) Naloxone reverses inhibitory effect of electroacupuncture on sympathetic cardiovascular reflex responses. *American Journal of Physiolology: Heart and Circulatory Physiology*, **276**: H2127–H2134.

Christensen, A.J., Wiebbe, J.S. and Lawton, W.J. (1997) Cynical hostility, powerful others control expectancies, and patient adherence in hemodialysis. *Psychosomatic Medicine*, 59: 307–312.

Christian, J.J. (1955) The effects of populations size on the adrenal glands of male mice in populations of fixed size. *American Journal of Physiology*, **185**: 292–300.

Cipher, D.J., Fernandez, E. and Clifford, P.A. (2002) Coping style influences compliance with multidisciplinary pain management. *Journal of Health Psychology*, **7**: 665–673.

Clukey, L. (2003) Anticipatory mourning: transitional processes of expected loss. *Dissertation Abstracts International: Section B: The Sciences and Engineering*, **63 (7-B)**: 3467.

Coan, R.M., Wong, G. and Coan, P.L. (1980) The acupuncture treatment of low back pain: a randomised controlled study. *American Journal of Chinese Medicine*, **8**: 181–189.

Coburn, E. and Sirois, W. (2001) A lifestyle how-to for night-shift nurses. *Nursing Management, Critical Care Choices Supplement*, **54**.

Cohen, S. and Wills, T.A. (1985) Stress, social support, and the buffering hypothesis. *Psychological Bulletin*, **98**: 310–357.

Cohen, S., Glass, D.C. and Singer, J.E. (1973) Apartment noise, auditory discrimination, and reading ability in children. *Journal of Experimental Social Psychology*, **9**: 407–422.

Cohen, S., Mermelstein, R., Kamarck, T. and Hoberman, H.N. (1985) Measuring the functional components of social support. In: *Social Support: Theory, Research, and Applications* (eds I.G. Sarason and B.R. Sarason). Martinus Nijhoff, Dordrecht: pp. 73–94.

Cohen, S., Tyrell, D. and Smith, A. (1993) Negative life events, perceived stress, negative affect, and susceptibility to the common cold. *Journal of Personality and Social Psychology*, **64**: 131–140.

Cohen, S., Frank, E. and Doyle, W.J. (1998) Types of stressors that increase susceptibility to the common cold in healthy adults. *Health Psychology*, **17**: 214–223.

Condon, L. (2001) Cruising for safer sex. *The Advocate*, **13 March**.

Cooper, C.L., Cooper, R.D. and Eaker, L.H. (1988) *Living with Stress*. Penguin, London.

Craik, F.I.M. and Lockhart, R. (1972) Levels of processing. *Journal of Experimental Psychology: General*, **104**: 268–294.

Cramer, J.A., Mattson, R.H., Prevey, M.L. *et al.* (1989) How often is medication taken as prescribed? *Journal of the American Medical Association*, **261**: 3273–3277.

Crawford, H.J. and Gruzelier, J.H. (1992) A midstream view of the neurophysiology of hypnosis: recent research and future directions. In: *Contemporary Hypnosis Research* (eds E. Fromm and M.R. Nash). Guilford Press, New York.

Crisson, J.E. and Keefe, F.J. (1988) The relationship of locus of control to pain coping strategies and psychological distress in chronic pain patients. *Pain*, **35**: 147–154.

Cunningham, M.R. (1979) Weather, mood, and helping behavior: quasi experiments with the sunshine Samaritan. *Journal of Personality and Social Psychology*, **37**: 1947–1956.

Curran, J.W., Morgan, W.M. and Hardy, A.M. (1985) The epidemiology of AIDS: current status and future prospects. *Science*, **229**: 1352–1357.

Daghio, M.M., Ciardullo, A.V., Cadiioli, T. *et al.* (2003) GPs' satisfaction with the doctor–patient encounter: findings from a community-based survey. *Family Practice*, **20**: 283–288.

Davis, C.B. (1989) The use of art therapy and group process with grieving children. *Issues in Comprehensive Pediatric Nursing*, **12**: 269–280.

De Craen, A.J.M., Roos, P.J., de Vries, A.L. and Kleijnen, J. (1996) Effect of colour of drugs: systematic review of perceived effect of drugs and of their effectiveness. *British Medical Journal*, **313**: 1624–1626.

DeLongis, A., Folkman, S. and Lazarus, R.S. (1988) The impact of daily stresses on health and mood: Psychological and social resources as mediators. *Journal of Personality and Social Psychology*, **54**: 486–495.

De Wit, J.B.F., Kok, G.J., Timmermans, C.A.M. and Wijnsma, P. (1990) Determinanten van veilig en condoomgerbruik bij jongeren. *Gedrag en Gezondheid*, **18**: 121–133.

Department of Health and Social Security (1998) *Our Healthier Nation: A contract for health*. Stationery Office, London.

DesCamp, K.D. and Thomas, C.C. (1993) Buffering nursing stress through play at work. *Western Journal of Nursing Research*, **15**: 619–627.

Deyo, R.A. and Inui, T.S. (1980) Dropouts and broken appointments: A literature review and agenda for future research. *Medical Care*, **18**: 1146–1157.

Diamond, E.G., Kittle, C.F. and Crickett, J.F. (1960) Comparison of internal mammary artery ligation and sham operation for angina pectoris. *American Journal of Cardiology*, **5**: 483–486.

DiMatteo, M.R. and DiNicola, D.D. (1982) *Achieving patient compliance: The psychology of the medical practitioner's role.* Pergamon, New York.

DiMatteo, M.R., Hays, R.D. and Prince, L.M. (1986) Relationship of physicians' nonvernal communication skills to patient satisfaction, appointment concompliance, and physician workload. *Health Psychology*, **5**: 581–594.

DiMatteo, M.R., Sherbourne, C.D., Hays, R.D. *et al.* (1993) Physicians' characteristics influence patients' adherence to medical treatment: results from the Medical Outcomes Study. *Health Psychology*, **12**: 93–102.

DiMatteo, M.R., Reiter, R.C. and Gambone, J.C. (1994) Enhancing medication adherence through communication and informed collaborative choice. *Health Communications*, **6**: 253–265.

DiNicola, D.D. and DiMatteo, M.R. (1984) Practitioners, patients, and compliance with medical regimens: a social psychological perspective. In: *Handbook of Psychology and Health*, vol. 4: *Social Psychological Aspects of Health* (eds A. Baum, S.E. Taylor and J.E. Singer). Laurence Erlbaum Associates, Hillsdale, NJ.

Doherty, W.J., Schrott, H.G., Metcalf, L. and Iasiello-Vailas, L. (1983) Effect of spouse support and health beliefs on medication adherence. *Journal of Family Practice*, **17**: 837–841.

Dohrenwend, B.P. (1973) Social status and stressful life events. *Journal of Personality and Social Psychology*, **28**: 225–235.

Dolce, J.J. (1987) Self-efficacy and disability beliefs in behavioural treatment of pain. *Behaviour and Research Therapies*, **25**: 289–299.

Donovan, J.L. and Blake, D.R. (1992) Patient non-compliance: deviance or reasoned decision-making? *Social Science and Medicine*, **34**: 507–513.

Dowson, D.I., Lewith, G.T. and Machin, D. (1985) The effects of acupuncture versus placebo in the treatment of headache. *Pain*, **21**: 35–42.

Duke, M.P. and Nowicki, S. (1972) Diagramming the shape of personal space: a new measure and social learning model for interpersonal distance. *Journal of Experimental Research in Personality*, **6**: 119–132.

Dunkel-Schetter, C. and Bennett, T.L. (1990) Differentiating the cognitive and behavioral aspects of social support. In: *Social Support: An international view* (eds B.R. Sarason, I.G. Sarason and G.R. Pierce). John Wiley, New York: pp. 267–296.

Dyregrov, K., Nordanger, D. and Dyregrov, A. (2003) Predictors of psychosocial stress after suicide, SIDS and accidents. *Death Studies*, **27**: 143–165.

Eagly, A.H. and Chaiken, S. (1993) *The Psychology of Attitudes*. Harcourt Brace Jovanovich, Fort Worth, TX.

Edelmann, R.J. (2000) *Psychosocial Aspects of the Health care Process*. Prentice Hall, Harlow, Essex.

Egan, G. (1986) *Exercises in Helping Skills*. Brookes Cole, Monterey, CA.

Elder, J.P., Sallis, J.F., Woodruff, S.I. and Widley, M.B. (1993) Tobacco-refusal skills and tobacco use among high-risk adolescents. *Journal of Behavioral Medicine*, **16**: 629–642.

Epping-Jordan, J.E. Compas, B.E. and Howell, D.C. (1994) Predictors of cancer progression in young adult men and women: avoidance, intrusive thoughts, and psychological symptoms. *Health Psychology*, **13**: 539–547.

Erlen, J.A., Riley, T.A. and Sereika, S.M. (1999) Psychometric properties of the Index of Homophobia Scale in registered nurses. *Journal of Nursing Measurement*, **7**: 117–133.

Evans, R.I. (1976) Smoking in children: developing a social-psychological strategy of deterrence. *Journal of Preventative Medicine*, **5**: 122–127.

Evans, G.W. (1979) Behavioral and physiological consequences of crowding in humans. *Journal of Applied Social Psychology*, **9**: 27–46.

Evans, P. (1998) Stress and coping. In: *The Psychology of Health: An introduction* (eds M. Pitts and K. Phillips). Routledge, London: pp. 47–67.

Evans, G.W., Jacobs, S.V., Dooley, D. and Catalano, R. (1987) The interaction of stressful life events and chronic strains on community mental health. *American Journal of Community Psychology*, **15**: 23–34.

Evans, R.I., Dratt, L.M., Raines, B.E. and Rosenberg, S.S. (1988) Social influences on smoking initiation: Importance of distinguishing descriptive versus mediating process variables. *Journal of Applied Social Psychology*, **18**: 925–943.

Evans, G.W., Hygge, S. and Bullinger, M. (1995) Chronic noise and psychological stress. *Psychological Science*, **6**: 333–338.

Eysenck, H.J. (1988) Personality, stress and cancer: prediction and prophylaxis. *British Journal of Medical Psychology*, **61**: 57–75.

Faulkner, A. (1995) *Working with Bereaved People*. Churchill Livingstone, Edinburgh.

Faust, J. and Melamed, B.G. (1984) Influence of arousal, previous experience, and age on surgery preparation of same day surgery and in-hospital pediatric patients. *Journal of Consulting and Clinical Psychology*, **52**: 359–365.

Feldman, P.E. (1956) The personal element in psychiatric research. *American Journal of Psychiatry*, **113**: 52–54.

Fenwick, R. and Tausig, M. (2000) Scheduling stress: family and health outcomes of shift work and schedule control. *American Behavioral Scientist*, **44**: 1179–1198.

Festinger, L. (1957) *A Theory of Cognitive Dissonance*. Stanford University Press, Stanford, CA.

Finney, J., Hook, R.J., Friman, P.C., Rapoff, M.A. and Christopherson, E.R. (1993) The over-estimation of adherence to pediatric medical regimens. *Children's Health Care*, **22**: 297–304.

Firth-Cozens, J. (1997) Predicting stress in general practitioners: 10 year follow up postal survey. *British Medical Journal*, **315**: 34–35.

Flay, B.R., Ockene, J.K. and Tager, I.B. (1992) Smoking: epidemiology, cessation and prevention. *Chest*, **102**: 277S–301S.

Folkman, S. Larazus, R.S., Gruen, R.J. and DeLongis, A. (1986) Appraising, coping, health status and psychological symptoms. *Journal of Personality and Social Psychology*, **50**: 571 579.

Fordyce, W.E. and Steger, J.C. (1979) Chronic pain. In: *Behavioral Medicine: Theory and practice* (eds O.F. Pomerleau and J.P. Brady). Williams & Wilkins, Baltimore, MD.

Forshaw, M. (2002) *Essential Health Psychology*. Arnold, London.

Forsythe, M., Calnan, M. and Wall, B. (1999) Doctors as patients: postal survey examining consultants and general practitioners' adherence to guidelines. *British Medical Journal*, **319**: 605–608.

Freeman, R., Lindner, R.L., Rooney, J. and Narendran, S. (2000) Dental students in Northern Ireland in 1992 and 1995: changing trends in psychological stress. *Stress Medicine*, **16**: 233–238.

Freud, S. (1894) The defence neuropsychoses. In: *The Standard Edition of the Complete Works of Sigmund Freud*, vol. 1 (ed. J. Strachey). Hogarth Press, London.

Freud, S. (1901) *The Psychopathology of Everyday Life*. Penguin, Harmondsworth.

Friedman, M. and Rosenman, R.H. (1974) *Type A Behavior and Your Heart*. Knopf, New York.

Frydenberg, E., Lewis, R., Kennedy, G. *et al.* (2003) Coping with concerns: an exploratory comparison of Australian, Colombian, German and Palestinian adolescents. *Journal of Youth and Adolescence*, **32**: 59–66.

Fuller, T.D., Edwards, J.N., Semsri, S. and Vorakitphokatorn, S. (1993) Housing, stress and physical well-being: evidence from Thailand. *Social Science and Medicine*, **36**: 1417–1428.

Galati, D., Scherer, K.R. and Ricci-Bitti, P.E. (1997) Voluntary facial expressions of emotion: Comparing congenitally blind with normally sighted encoders. *Journal of Personality and Social Psychology*, **73**: 1363–1379.

Garner, D.M., Garfinkel, P.E., Schwartz, D. and Thompson, M. (1980) Cultural expectations of thinness in women. *Psychological Reports*, **47**: 483–491.

Gass, K.A. (1989) Appraisal, coping and resources: markers associated with the health of aged widow and widowers. In: *Older Bereaved Spouses* (ed. D.A. Lund). Hemisphere Publishing, New York.

Gastorf, J.W. and Galanos, A.N. (1983) Patient compliance and physicians attitude. *Family Practice Research Journal*, **2**: 190–198.

Gefland, S., Ulman, L.P. and Krasner, L. (1963) The placebo-response – an experimental approach. *Journal of Nervous and Mental Diseases*, **136**: 379–387.

Gerber, L., Rusalem, R. and Hannon, N. (1975) Anticipatory grief and aged widows and widowers. *Journal of Gerontology*, **30**: 225–229.

Gibbs, S., Waters, W.E. and George, C.F. (1987) The design of prescription information leaflets and the feasibility of their use in general practice. *Pharmaceutical Medicine*, **2**: 23–33.

Gibbs, S., Waters, W.E. and George, C.F. (1989) The benefits of prescription information leaflets (1). *British Journal of Clinical Pharmacology*, **27**: 723–739.

Gibbs, S., Waters, W.E. and George, C.F. (1990) Communicating information to patients about medicine. Prescription information leaflets: a national survey. *Journal of the Royal Society of Medicine*, **83**: 292–297.

Gibson, D.R. (2001) Effectiveness of syringe exchange programs in reducing HIV risk behavior and HIV seroconversion among injecting drug users. *AIDS*, **15**: 1329–1341.

Gilbar, O. (1989) Who refuses chemotherapy: a profile. *Psychological Reports*, **64**: 1291–1297.

Glasgow, R.E., McCaul, K.D. and Schafer, L.C. (1986) Barriers to regimen adherence among persons with insulin-dependent diabetes. *Journal of Behavioral Medicine*, **9**: 65–77.

Glick, I.O., Weiss, R.S. and Parkes, C.M. (1974) *The First Year of Bereavement*. John Wiley, New York.

Goldberg, E.L. and Comstock, G.W. (1976) Life events and subsequent illness. *American Journal of Epidemiology*, **104**: 146–158.

Goodall, T.A. and Halford, W.K. (1991) Self-management of diabetes mellitus: a critical review. *Health Psychology*, **10**: 1–8.

Gowdey, C.W. (1983) A guide to the pharmacology of placebos. *Canadian Medical Association Journal*. **128**: 921–925.

Gracely, R.H., Dubner, R., Deeter, W.R. and Wolskee, P.J. (1985) Clinical expectations influence placebo analgesia. *Lancet*, **1**: 43.

Greene, M.G., Adelman, R., Charon, R. and Hoffman, S. (1986) Ageism in the medical encounter: an exploratory study of the language and behavior of doctors with their old and young patients. *Language and Communication*, **6**: 113–124.

Guadagnoli, E. and Ward, P. (1998) Patient participation in decision-making. *Social Science and Medicine*, **47**: 329–339.

Haas, H., Fink, H. and Hartfelder, G. (1959) Das Placeboproblem. *Forschritte der Arzneimittelforschung*, **1**: 279–354.

Hadlow, J. and Pitts, M. (1991) The understanding of common health terms by doctors, nurses and patients. *Social Science and Medicine*, **32**: 193–196.

Haefner, D. and Kirscht, J. (1970) Motivational and behavioral effects of modifying beliefs, *Public Health Reports*, **58**: 478–484.

Hall, J.A. and Dornan, M.C. (1988a) Meta-analysis of satisfaction with medical care: Description of research domain and analysis of overall satisfaction levels. *Social Science and Medicine*, **27**: 737–644.

Hall, J.A. and Dornan, M.C. (1988b) What patients like about their medical care and how often they are asked. *Social Science and Medicine*, **27**: 935–939.

Hall, J.A. and Dornan, M.C. (1990) Patient socio-demographic characteristics as predictors of satisfaction with medical care: a meta-analysis. *Social Science and Medicine*, **30**: 811–818.

Hall, J.A., Roter, D.L. and Katz, N.R. (1988) meta-analysis correlates of provider behavior in medical encounters. *Medical Care*, **26**: 657–675.

Hamburg, B.A. and Inoff, G.E. (1982) Relationship between behavioural factors and diabetic control in diabetic control in children and adolescents: a camp study. *Psychosomatic Medicine*, **44**: 321–329.

Harlan, L.C., Bernstein, A.M. and Kesler, L.G. (1991) Cervical cancer screening: who is not screened and why? *American Journal of Public Health*, **81**: 885–890.

Harris, L. (1999) Irritable bowel syndrome and stress. *Gut Reaction: The Journal of the IBS Network*, **34**: 6.

Harris, L. and associates (1980) *The Steelcase National Study of Office Environments, II: Comfort and Productivity in the Office of the 80s*. Steelcase, Inc., Grand Rapids, MI.

Harwood, A. (1971) The hot-cold theory of disease: implications for treatment of Puerto Rican patients. *Journal of the American Medical Association*, **216**: 1153–1158.

Haynes, R.B. (1976) A critical review of the 'determinants' of patient compliance with therapeutic regimens. In: *Compliance with Therapeutic Regimens* (eds D.L. Sackett and R.B. Haynes). Johns Hopkins University Press, Baltimore, MD: pp. 26–39.

Haynes, R.B. (1979) Determinants of compliance: the disease and the mechanics of treatment. In: *Compliance in Health Care* (eds R.B. Haynes, D.W. Tayor and D.L. Sakett). Johns Hopkins University Press, Baltimore, MD.

Haynes, R.B., Taylor, D.W., Sackett, D.L. *et al.* (1980) Can simple clinical measurements detect non-compliance? *Hypertension*, **2**: 757–764.

Haynes, R.B., Wang, E. and de Mota Gomes, M. (1987) A critical review of interventions to improve compliance with prescribed medication. *Patient Education and Counselling*, **10**: 155–166.

Hays, R.D., Kravitz, R.L., Mazel, R.M. *et al.* (1994) The impact of patient adherence on health outcomes for patients with chronic disease in the Medical Outcomes Study. *Journal of Behavioral Medicine*, **17**: 347–360.

Hegel, M.T., Ayllon, T., Thiel, G. and Oulton, B. (1992) Improving adherence to fluid restrictions in male haemodialysis patients: a comparison of cognitive and behavioral approaches. *Health Psychology*, **11**: 324–330.

Helman, C.G. (1994) *Culture, Health and Illness: An introduction for health professionals*. Butterworth-Heinemann, Oxford.

Helmstetter, F.J. and Bellgowan, P.S. (1994) Hypoalgesia in response to sensitization during acute noise stress. *Behavioral Neuroscience*, **108**: 177–185.

Herbert, T.B. and Cohen, S. (1993) Stress and immunity in humans: a meta-analytic review. *Psychonomic Medicine*, **55**: 364–379.

Hinkley, J.J., Craig, H.K. and Anderson, L.A. (1990) Communication characteristics of provider-patient information exchanges. In: *Handbook of Language and Social Psychology* (eds H. Giles and W.P. Robinson). John Wiley, Chichester.

Hochbaum, G.M. (1958) *Public Participation in medical screening programmes: a sociopsychological study*. Public Health Service Publication 572. US Government Printing Office, Washington DC.

Hodgson, C.J.R. (2001) Health locus of control, perception of risk and risk-taking behaviour in older adolescents. Dissertation Abstracts International: Section B, **61(9-B)**: 4650.

Holmes, T.H. and Rahe, R.H. (1967) The social readjustment rating scale. *Journal of Psychosomatic Research*, **11**: 213–218.

Holroyd, K.A. and Penzien, D.B. (1990) Pharmacological versus non-pharmacological prophylaxis of recurrent migraine headache: a meta-analytic review of clinical trials. *Pain*, **42**: 1–13.

Hooper, E.M., Comstock, L.M., Goodwin, J.M. and Goodwin, J.S. (1982) Patient characteristics that influence physician behavior. *Medical Care*, **20**: 630–638.

Horne, R. and Weinman, J. (2002) Self-regulation and self-management in asthma: exploring the role of illness perceptions and treatment beliefs in explaining non-adherence to preventer medication. *Psychology and Health*, **17**: 17–32.

Horowitz, R.I. and Horowitz, S.M. (1993) Adherence to treatment and health outcomes. *Archives of Internal Medicine*, **153**: 1863–1868.

House, J.S., Robbins, C. and Metzner, H.L. (1982) The association of social relationships and activities with mortality: prospective evidence from the Tecumseh Community Health Study. *American Journal of Epidemiology*, **116**: 123–140.

Houts, P.S., Bachrach, R., Witmer, J.T., Tringali, C.A., Bucher, J.A. and Localio, R.A. (1998) Using pictographs to enhance recall of spoken medical instructions. *Patient Education and Counselling*, **35**: 83–88.

Howard, D.J. (1997) Familiar phrases as peripheral peripheral persuasion cue. *Journal of Experimental Social Psychology*, **33**: 231–243.

Hrobjartsson, A. and Gotzche, P.C. (2001) Is the placebo powerless? An analysis of clinical trials comparing placebo with no treatment. *New England Journal of Medicine*, **344**: 1594–1602.

Hui, K.S., Liu, J., Makris, N. *et al.* (2000) Acupuncture modulates the limbic system and subcortical gray structures of the human brain: evidence from fMRI studies in normal subjects. *Human Brain Mapping*, **9**: 13–25.

Huntingdon, D. (1987) *Social Skills and General Medical Practice.* Allen & Unwin, London.

Insel, P.M. and Roth, W.T. (1996) *Core Concepts in Health.* Mayfield, London.

International Association for the Study of Pain Subcommittee on Taxonomy (1979). Pain terms: a list with definitions and notes on usage. *Pain*, **6**: 99–102.

Inui, T.S., Carter, W.B. and Pecoraro, R.E. (1981) Screening for non-compliance among patients with hypertension: is self-report the best available measure? *Medical Care*, **19**: 1061–1064.

Ising, H. and Melchert, H.U. (1980) Endocrine and cardiovascular effects of noise. In: *Noise as a Public Health Problem: Proceedings of the Third International Congress.* (ASHA Report no. 10). American Speech and Hearing Association, Rockville, MD: pp. 194–203.

Jackson, R.L., Maier, S.F. and Coon, D.J. (1979) Long-term analgesic effects of inescapable shock and learned helplessness. *Science*, **206**: 91–93.

Jacobs, S. (1999) *Traumatic Grief: Diagnosis, treatment, and prevention.* Brunner/Mazel, Philadelphia, PA.

Jamner, L.D. and Tursky, B. (1987) Syndrome-specific descriptor profiling: a psychophysiological and psychophysical approach, *Health Psychology*, **6**: 417–430.

Janis, I.L. and Feshbach, S. (1953) Effects of fear-arousing communications. *Journal of Abnormal and Social Psychology*, **48**: 78–92.

Janis, I.L. and Field, P.B. (1959) A behavioral assessment of persuasibility: consistency of individual differences. In: *Personality and Persuasibility* (eds C.I. Hovland and I.L. Janis). Yale University Press, New Haven, CN: pp. 29–54.

Janis, I.L. and Hovland, C.I. (1959) An overview of persuasibility research. In: *Personality and Persuasibility* (eds C.I. Hovland and I.L. Janis). Yale University Press, New Haven, CN: pp. 1–26.

Janssen, M., De Wit, J., Stroebe, W. and van Griensven, F. (1998) Socio-economic status and risk of HIV in young gay men. Unpublished manuscript, University of Utrecht, Utrecht.

Jasper, M. (2003) *Beginning Reflective Practice*. Nelson Thornes, Cheltenham.

Jeffery, R. (1979) Normal rubbish: deviant patients in casualty departments. *Sociology of Health and Illness*, **1**: 90–108.

Jones, J.W. and Bogat, A. (1978) Air pollution and human aggression. *Psychological Reports*, **43**: 721–722.

Kabat-Zin, J. and Chapman-Waldrop, A. (1988) Compliance with an outpatient stress reduction program: rates and predictors of program completion. *Journal of Behavioral Medicine*, **11**: 333–352.

Kalichman, S., Stein, J.A., Malow, R. *et al.* (2002) Predicting protected sexual behaviour using the Information–Motivation–Behaviour skills model among adolescent substance abusers in court-ordered treatment. *Psychology, Health and Medicine*, **7**: 327–338.

Kaplan, R.M. and Simon, H.J. (1990) Compliance in medical care: reconsideration of self-predictions. *Annals of Behavioral Medicine*, 12: 66–71.

Karasek, R.A., Baker, D., Marxer, F. *et al.* (1981) Job decision latitude, job demands and cardiovascular disease: a prospective study of Swedish men. *American Journal of Public Health*. **71**: 694–705.

Karasek, R.A., Theorell, T., Schwartz, J. *et al.* (1988) Job characteristics in relation to the prevalence of myocardial infarction in the US Health Examination Survey (HES) and the Health and Nutrition Examination Survey (HANES). *American Journal of Public Health*, **78**: 910–918.

Karoly, P. (1985) *Measurement Strategies in Health Psychology*. John Wiley, New York.

Keefe, F.J. and Block, A.R. (1982) Development of an observation method for assessing pain behavior in chronic low back pain patients. *Behavior Therapy*, **13**: 363–375.

Keller, S.E., Shifflett, S.C., Schleifer, S.J. and Bartlett, J.A. (1994) Stress, immunity, and health. In: *Handbook of Human Stress and Immunity* (eds R. Glaser and J.K. Kiecolt-Glaser). Academic Press, San Diego, CA: pp. 217–244.

Kelley, A.J. (1979) A media role for public health compliance? In: *Compliance in Health Care* (eds R.B. Hayes, D.W. Taylor and D.L. Sackett). Johns Hopkins University Press, Baltimore, MD.

Kelly, J.A., St Lawrence, J.S., Brasfield, T.L. and Hood, H.V. (1989) Behavioral intervention to reduce AIDS risk activities. *Journal of Counselling and Clinical Psychology*, **57**: 60–67.

Kelly, J.A., St Lawrence, J.S., Brasfield, T.L. *et al.* (1990) Psychological factors that predict AIDS high-risk versus AIDS precautionary behavior. *Journal of Consulting and Clinical Psychology*, **58**: 117–120.

Kerr, J., Engel, J., Schlesinger-Raab, A., Sauer, H. and Holzel, D. (2003) Doctor–patient communication: results of a four-year prospective study in rectal cancer patients. *Diseases of the Colon and Rectum*, **46**: 1038–1046.

Keys, A., Brozek, J., Henschel, A. *et al.* (1950) *The Biology of Human Starvation*. University of Minnesota Press, Minneapolis, MN.

Kiecolt-Glaser, J.K. and Glaser, R. (1986) Psychological influences on immunity. *Psychosomatics*, **27**: 621–624.

Kiecolt-Glaser, J.K., Glaser, R., Dyer, C. *et al.* (1987) Chronic stress and immune function in family caregivers of Alzheimer's disease victims. *Psychosomatic Medicine*, **49**: 523–535.

Kiecolt-Glaser, J.K., Dyer, C.S. and Shuttleworth, E.C. (1988) Upsetting social interactions and distress among Alzheimer's disease family caregivers: a replication and extension. *American Journal of Community Psychology*, **16**: 825–837.

Kiecolt-Glaser, J.K., Malarkey, W.B., Cacioppo, J.T. and Glaser, R. (1994) Stressful personal relationships: Immune and endocrine function. In: *Handbook of human stress and immunity* (eds R. Glaser and J.K. Kiecolt-Glaser). Academic Press, San Diego, CA: pp. 321–339.

Kiernan, P.J. and Issacs, J.B. (1981) Use of drugs by the elderly. *Journal of the Royal Society of Medicine*, **74**: 196–200.

Kirsch, I., Montgomery, G. and Sapirstein, G. (1995) Hypnosis as an adjunct to cognitve-behavioral therapy: a meta-analysis. *Journal of Consulting and Clinical Psychology*, **63**: 214–220.

Kirscht, J.P., Becker, M., Haefner, D. and Maiman, L. (1978) Effects of threatening communications and mothers' health beliefs on weight change in obese children. *Journal of Behavioral Medicine*, **1**: 147–157.

Kittel, F., Kornitzer, M., Draimaix, M. and Beriot, I. (1993) Health behavior in Belgian studies: Who is doing best? Paper presented at the European Congress of Psychology, Tampere, Finland.

Klenerman, L., Slade, P.D., Stanley, I.M. *et al.* (1995) The prediction of chronicity in patients with an acute attack of low back pain in general practice setting. *Spine*, **20**: 478–484.

Kobasa, S.C. (1979) Stressful life events and health: an enquiry into hardiness. *Journal of Personality and Social Psychology*, **37**: 1–11.

Koehler, T., Thiede, G. and Thoens, M. (2002) Long and short-term forgetting of word associations. An experimental study of the Freudian concepts of resistance and repression. *Zeitschrift für Klinische Psychologie, Psychiatrie und Psychotherapie*, **50**: 328–333.

Korsch, B.M. and Negrete, V. (1972) Doctor–patient communication. *Scientific American*, **227**: 66–74.

Koski-Jannes, A. (1994) Drinking-related locus of control as a predictor of drinking after treatment. *Addictive Behaviors*, **19**: 491–495.

Kravitz, R.L., Hays, R.D., Sherbourne, C.D. *et al.* (1993) Recall of recommendations and adherence to advice among patients with chronic medical conditions. *Archives of Internal Medicine*, **153**: 1869–1878.

Krebs, J.R. and Davies, N.B. (1993) *An Introduction to Behavioural Ecology*. Blackwell, Oxford.

Krechowiecka, I. (2001) Tomorrow's World: interactive exhibits. *Guardian*, **26 June**: 5.

Krokosky, N.J. and Reardon, R.C. (1989) The accuracy of nurses' and doctors' perception of patient pain. In: *Key Aspects of Comfort: Management of pain, fatigue and nausea* (eds S.G. Fuk, E.M. Tornquist, M.T. Champagne *et al.*). Springer, New York: pp. 127–140.

Kroeber, A.L. (1948) *Anthropology*. Harcourt, New York.

Kübler-Ross, E. (1969) *On Death and Dying*. Macmillan, New York.

Laforge, R.G., Greene, G.W. and Prochaska, J.O. (1994) Psychosocial factors influencing low fruit and vegetable consumption. *Journal of Behavioral Medicine*, **17**: 361–374.

Langenfeld, M.C. (2000) The effects of hypnosis on pain-control with people living with HIV-AIDS. *Dissertation Abstracts International: Section B: The Sciences and Engineering*, **60**(II-B): 5780.

Langer, E.J. and Rodin, J. (1976) The effects of choice and enhances personal responsibility for the aged: a field experiment in an institutional setting. *Journal of Personality and Social Psychology*, **34**: 191–198.

Lazarus, R.S. and Folkman, S. (1984) *Stress, Appraisal, and Coping*. Springer-Verlag, New York.

Leedham, B., Meyerowitz, B.E., Muirhead, J. and Frist, W.H. (1995) Positive expectations predict health after heart transplantation. *Health Psychology*, **13**: 74–79.

Lennon, M.C., Martin, J.L. and Dean, L. (1990) The influence of social support on AIDS-related grief reaction among gay men. *Social Science and Medicine*, **31**: 477–484.

Lent, R.W., Crimmings, A.M. and Russell, R.K. (1981) Subconscious reconditioning: evaluation of a placebo strategy for outcome. *Behaviour Research and Therapy*, **12**: 138–143.

Lepore, S.J., Evans, G.W. and Schneider, M.L. (1991) Dynamic role of social support in the link between chronic stress and psychological distress. *Journal of Personality and Social Psychology*, **61**: 899–909.

Lercher, P., Hortnagel, J. and Kofler, W.W. (1993) Work noise, annoyance and blood pressure: Combined effects with stressful working conditions. *International Archives of Occupational and Environmental Health*, **65**: 23–28.

Letham, J., Slade, P.D., Troup, J.D.G. and Bentley, G. (1983) Outline of a fear-avoidance model of exaggerated pain perception. Part 1. *Behavioural Research Therapy*, **21**: 401–408.

Leventhal, H. (1970) Findings and theory in the study of fear communications. *Advances in Experimental Social Psychology*, **5**: 119–186.

Leventhal, H. and Cleary, P.D. (1980) The smoking problem: a review of the research and theory in behavioural risk moderation. *Psychological Bulletin*, **88**. 370–405.

Levine, J.D., Gordon, N.C. and Fields, H.L. (1979) The role of endorphins in placebo analgesia. In: *Advances in Pain Research and Therapy*, vol. 3 (eds J.J. Bonica, J.C. Liebeskind and D. Albe-Fessard). Raven Press, New York.

Lewis, T., Osborn, L.M., Lewis, K. *et al.* (1988) Influence of parental knowledge and opinions on 12-month diphtheria, tetanus, and pertussis vaccination rates. *American Journal of Diptheria C*, **142**: 283–286.

Ley, P. (1972) Primacy, rated importance and the recall of medical information. *Journal of Health and Social Behavior*, **13**: 331–337.

Ley, P. (1979) Memory for medical information. *British Journal of Social and Clinical Psychology*, **18**: 245–256.

Ley, P. (1981) Professional non-compliance: a neglected problem. *British Journal of Clinical Psychology*, **20**: 151–154.

Ley, P. (1982) Studies of recall in medical settings. *Human Learning*, **1**: 223–233.

Ley, P. (1988) *Communicating with Patients*. Croom Helm, London.

Ley, P. and Llewelyn, S. (1995) Improving patients' understanding, recall, satisfaction and compliance. In: *Health Psychology: Processes and applications* (eds A. Broome and S. Llewelyn). Chapman & Hall, London: pp. 75–98.

Ley, P., Jain, V.K. and Skilbeck, C.E. (1975) A method for decreasing patients' medication errors. *Psychological Medicine*, **6**: 599–601.

Liberman, R. (1962) An analysis of the placebo phenomenon. *Journal of Chronic Diseases*, **15**: 761–783.

Lin, N., Simeone, R.S., Ensel, W.M. and Kuo, W. (1979) Social support, stressful life events, and illness: a model and an empirical test. *Journal of Health and Social Behaviour*, **20**: 108–119.

Lipton, J.A. and Marbach, J.J. (1984) Ethnicity and the pain experience. *Social Science and Medicine*,**19**: 1279–1298.

Loeser, J.D. (1989) Chronic pain. In: *Issues in Behavioural Medicine* (eds F.C. Seitz, J.E. Carr and M. Covey). Clinical Management Consultants, Bozeman, MT.

Longshore, D., Blunthenthalm, R.N. and Stein, M.D. (2001) Needle exchange program attendance and injection risk in Providence, Rhode Island. *AIDS Education and Prevention*, **13(1)**: 78–90.

Lorenc, L. and Branthwaite, A. (1993) Are older adults less compliant with prescribed medication than younger adults? *British Journal of Clinical Psychology*, **32**: 485–492.

Lutz, R.W., Silbret, M. and Olshan, W. (1983) Treatment outcome and compliance with therapeutic regimens: Long-term follow-up of a multidisciplinary pain program. *Pain*, **17**: 301–308.

Lynch, D.J., Birk, T.J., Weaver, M.T. *et al.* (1992) Adherence to exercise interventions in the treatment of hypercholesterolemia. *Journal of Behavior Medicine*, **15**: 365–377.

Macarthur, C., Saunders, N., and Feldman, W. (1995) *Heliobacter pylori*, gastroduodenal diease, and recurrent abdominal pain in children. *Journal of the American Medical Asssociation*, **273**: 729–734.

McAlister, A.L., Perry, C., Killen, J. *et al.* (1980) Pilot study of smoking, alcohol, and drug abuse prevention. *American Journal of Public Health*, **70**: 719–721.

McAuley, E. (1993) Self-efficacy and the maintenance of exercise participation in older adults. *Journal of Behavioral Medicine*, **16**: 103–113.

McAvoy, B.R. and Raza, R. (1988) Asian women: (i) Contraceptive knowledge, attitudes and usage, (ii) Contraceptive services and cervical cytology. *Health Trends*, **20**: 11–17.

McCaul, K.D., Dyche Bransetter, A., Schroder, D.M. and Glasgow, R.M. (1996) What is the relationship between breast cancer risk and mammography screening? A meta-analytic review. *Health Psychology*, **15**: 423–429.

McKinlay, J.B. (1975) Who is really ignorant – physician or patient? *Journal of Health and Social Behaviour*, **16**: 3–11.

McCulluch, D.K., Mitchell, R.D., Ambler, J. and Tattersall, R.B. (1983) Influence of imaginative teaching of diet on compliance and metabolic control in insulin dependent diabetes. *British Medical Journal*, **287**: 1858–1861.

McDougall, G.J. (1993) Therapeutic issues with gay and lesbian elders. *Clinical Gerontologist*, **14**: 45–57.

McGowan, L.P.A., Clarke-Carter, D.D. and Pitts, M.K. (1998) Chronic pelvic pain: a meta-analytic review. *Psychology and Health*, **13**: 937–951.

McGrady, A. (1994) Effects of group relaxation training and thermal biofeedback on blood pressure and related physiological and psychological variables in essential hypertension. *Biofeedback and Self*, **19**: 51–66.

McGuire, W.J. (1968) Personality and attitude change: a theoretical housing. In: *Psychological Foundations of Attitudes* (eds A.G. Greenwald, T.C. Brock and T.M. Ostrom). Academic Press, New York.

McGuire, W.J. (1969) The nature of attitudes and attitude change. In: *Handbook of Social Psychology*, 2nd edn (eds G. Lindzey and E. Aronson). Addison-Wesley, Reading, MA: vol. 3, pp. 136–314.

MacKinnon, D.P. and Fenaughty, A.M. (1993) Substance use and memory for health warning labels. *Health Psychology*, **12**: 147–150.

Macleod Clark, J. (1982) Nurse/patient verbal interaction. Royal College of Nursing, Steinberg Collection, London.

Manning, M.M. and Wright, T.L. (1983) Self-efficacy expectancies, outcome expectancies and the persistence of pain control in childbirth. *Journal of Personality and Social Psychology*, **45**: 421–431.

Manstead, A.S.R., Proffitt, C. and Smart, J.L. (1983) Predicting and understanding mothers' infant-feeding intentions and behavior: testing the theory of reasoned action. *Journal of Personality and Social Psychology*, **44**: 657–671.

Manuck, S.B., Kaplan, J.R. and Matthews, K.A. (1986) Behavioral antecedents of coronary heart disease and atherosclerosis. *Atherosclerosis*, **6**: 1–14.

Marks, D.F., Murray, M., Evans, B. and Willig, C. (2000) *Health Psychology: Theory, Research and Practice*. Sage, London.

Marshall, J.R. and Funch, D.P. (1986) Gender and illness behaviour among colorectal cancer patients. *Women and Health*, **11**: 67–82.

Martin, J.L. (1988) Psychological consequences of AIDS-related bereavement among gay men. *Journal of Consulting and Clinical Psychology*, **56**: 856–862.

Martin, S.C., Arnold, R.M. and Parker, R.M. (1988) Gender and medical socialization. *Journal of Health and Social Behavior*, **29**: 333–343.

Marucha, P.T., Kiecolt Glaser, J.K. and Favagehi, M. (1998) Mucosal wound healing is impaired by examination stress. *Psychosomatic Medicine*, **60**: 362–365.

Maschke, C., Ising, H. and Arndt, D. (1995) Nachtlicher Verkehrslarm und Gesundheit. *Bundesgesund Heilsblatt*, **38**: 130–136.

Mason, E. (1970) Obesity in pet dogs. *Veterinary Record*, **86**: 612–616.

Masur, F.T. III (1981) Adherence to health care regimens. In: *Medical Psychology: Contributions to Behavioral Medicine* (eds C.K. Prokop and L.A. Bradley). Academic Press, New York.

Mathews, K.E. and Canon, L.K. (1975) Environmental noise level as a determinant of helping behavior. *Journal of Personality and Social Psychology*, **32**: 571–577.

Matsumoto, D. and Ekman, P. (1989) American–Japanese cultural differences in intensity ratings of facial expressions of emotion. *Motivation and Emotion*, **13**: 143–57.

Matthews, S.C., Camacho, A., Mills, P.J. and Dimsdale, J.E. (2003) The Internet for medical information about cancer: help or hindrance. *Psychosomatics: Journal of Consultation Liaison Psychiatry*, **44**: 100–103.

Meeuweesen, L., Schaap, C. and Van der Staak, C. (1991) Verbal analysis of doctor–patient communication. *Social Science and Medicine*, **32**: 1143–1150.

Meichenbaum, D.H. and Turk, D.C. (1987) *Facilitating Treatment Adherence: A practitioner's guidebook*. Plenum Press, New York.

Melzack, R. (1973) *The Puzzle of Pain*. Basic Books, New York.

Melzack, R. (1975) McGill Pain Questionnaire: major properties and scoring methods. *Pain*, **1**: 277–299.

Melzack, R. (1993) Pain: Past, present and future. *Canadian Journal of Experimental Psychology*, **47**: 615–629.

Melzack, R. and Wall, P.D. (1965) Pain mechanisms: a new theory. *Science*, **150**: 971–979.

Melzack, R. and Wall, P.D. (1982) *The Challenge of Pain*. Basic Books, New York.

Meszaros, J.R., Asch, D.A., Baron, J. *et al.* (1996) Cognitive processes and the decisions of some parents to forego pertussis vaccination for their children. *Journal of Clinical Epidemiology*, **59**: 697–703.

Michie, S., Marteau, T.M. and Kidd, J. (1992) Predicting antenatal class attendance: Attitudes of self and others. *Psychology and Health*, **7**: 225–234.

Miller, M., Eskild, A., Mella, I. *et al.* (2001) Gender differences in syringe exchange program use in Oslo, Norway. *Addiction*, **96**: 1639–1651.

Miller-Johnson, S., Emery, R.E., Marvin, R.S., Clarke, W., Lovinger, R. and Marin, M. (1994) Parent–child relationships and management of insulin-dependent diabetes mellitus. *Journal of Consulting and Clinical Psychology*, **62**: 603–610.

Milot, J. and Rosental, R.A. (1967) *Experiential Effects in Behavioural Research*. Appleton-Century Crofts, New York.

Monane, M., Bohn, R.L., Gurvitz, J.H., Glynn, R.J., Levin, R. and Avorn, J. (1996) Compliance with antihypertensive therapy among elderly Medicaid enrolees: the rates of age, gender and race. *American Journal of Public Health*, **86**: 1805–1808.

Montano, D.E. and Taplin, S.H. (1991) A test of an expanded theory of reasoned action to predict mammography participation. *Social Science and Medicine*, **32**: 733–741.

Montgomery, G.H., DuHamel, K.N. and Redd, W.H. (2000) A meta-analysis of hypnotically induced analgesia: how effective is hypnosis? *International Journal of Clinical and Experimental Hypnosis*, **48**: 138–153.

Morisky, D. (1983) Five-year blood pressure control and mortality following health education for hypertensive patients. *American Journal of Public Health*, **73**: 153–162.

Morrison, A.F., Kline, F.G. and Miller, P. (1976) Aspects of adolescent information acquisition about drugs and alcohol topics. In: *Communication Research and Drug Education* (ed. R. Ortman). Sage, Beverly Hills, CA.

Murdock, B.B. (1962) The serial position effect of free recall, *Journal of Experimental Psychology*, **64**: 482–488.

Murray, M. and McMillan, C. (1993) Health beliefs, locus of control, emotional control and women's cancer screening behaviour. *British Journal of Clinical Psychology*, **32**: 87–100.

Nagy, M.H. (1948) The child's theories concerning death. *Journal of Genetic Psychology*, **73**: 3–27.

Nakao, M., Nomura, S., Shimosawa, T. *et al.* (1997) Clinical effects of blood pressure biofeedback treatment on hypertension by auto-shaping. *Psychosomatic Medicine*, **59**: 331–338.

New, S.J. and Senior, M. (1991) 'I don't believe in needles': qualitative aspects of study into the uptake of infant immunisation in two English health authorities. *Social Science and Medicine*, **33**: 509–518.

Newmeyer, J.A., Feldman, H.W., Biernacki, P. and Watters, J.K. (1989) Preventing AIDS contagion among intravenous drug users. In: *The AIDS Pandemic: A global emergency* (ed. R. Bolton). Gordon & Breach, New York: pp. 75–83.

Ng, B., Dimsdale, J.E., Shragg, G.P. and Deutsch, R. (1996) Ethnic differences in analgesic consumption for post-operative pain. *Psychosomatic Medicine*, **58**: 125–129.

Nolen-Hoeksema, S. and Larson, J. (1999) *Coping with Loss*. Lawrence Erlbaum, Mahwah, NJ.

Norman, N.M. and Tedeschi, J.T. (1989) Self-presentation, reasoned action, and adolescents' decisions to smoke cigarettes. *Journal of Applied Social Psychology*, **19**: 543–558.

Norman, P., Bennett, P., Smith, C. and Murphy, S. (1998) Health locus of control and health behaviour. *Journal of Health Psychology*, **3**: 171–180.

Norman, P., Searle, A., Harrad, R. and Vedhara, K. (2003) Predicting adherence to eye-patching in children with amblyopia: an application of protection motivation theory. *British Journal of Health Psychology*, **8**: 67–82.

Novelli, P. (1997) Knowledge about causes of peptic ulcer disease – United States, March–April 1997. *Morbidity and Mortality Weekly Reports*, **46**: 985–987.

Oakley, A. (1980) *Women Confined*. Martin Robertson, Oxford.

Oakley, D., Alden, P. and Degun Mather, M. (1996) The use of hypnosis in therapy with adults. *Psychologist*, **9**: 502–505.

O'Brien, M.K. (1997) Compliance among health professionals. In: *Cambridge Handbook of Psychology, Health and Medicine* (eds A. Baum, S. Newman, J. Weinman, R. West and C. McManus). Cambridge University Press, Cambridge.

O'Brien, S. and Lee, L. (1990) Effects of videotape intervention on Pap smear knowledge, attitudes and behavior. *Behaviour Changes*, **7**: 143–150.

O'Carroll, R.E., Smith, K.B., Grubb, N.R. *et al.* (2001) Psychological factors associated with delay in attending hospital following a myocardial infarction. *Journal of Psychosomatic Research*, **51**: 611–614.

Ogden, J., Branson, R., Bryett, A. *et al.* (2003) What's in a name? An experimental study of patients' views of the impact and function of a diagnosis. *Family Practice*, **20**: 248–253.

Ong, L.M.L., deHaes, J.C.J.M., Hoos, A.M. and Lammes, F.B. (1995) Doctor–patient communication: a review of the literature. *Social Science and Medicine*, **40**: 903–918.

Orme, C.M. and Binik, Y.M. (1989) Consistency of adherence across regimen demands. *Health Psychology*, **8**: 27–43.

Page, R. (1977) Noise and helping behavior. *Environment and Behavior*, **9**: 311–314.

Page, B., Chitwood, D.D., Prince, P.C. *et al.* (1990) Intraveous drug use and HIV infection in Miami. *Medical Anthropology Quarterly* (New Series), **4**: 56–71.

Pagoto, S., McCharguc, D. and Fuqua, R.W. (2003) Effects of a multicomponent intervention on motivation and sun protection behavior among Midwestern beachgoers. *Health Psychology*, **22**: 429–433.

Paran, E., Amir, M. and Yaniv, N. (1996) Evaluating the response of mild hypertensives to biofeedback-assisted relaxation using a mental stress test. *Journal of Behavior Therapy and Experimental Psychiatry*, **27**: 157–167.

Park, L.C. and Covi, L. (1965) Nonblind placebo trial. *Archives of General Psychiatry*, **12**: 336–345.

Parkes, C.M. (1972) *Bereavement: Studies of grief in adult life*. International Universities Press, New York.

Parkes, C.M. (1975) Determinants of grief following bereavement. *Omega*, **6**: 303–323.

Parkes, C.M. (1980) Terminal care: an evaluation of an advisory domiciliary service at St Christopher's Hospice. *Postgraduate Medical Journal*, **56**: 685–689.

Parkes, C.M. (2000) Bereavement as a psychosocial transition: processes of adaptation to change. In: *Death, Dying and Bereavement* (eds D. Dickenson, M. Johnson and J.S. Katz). Sage/Open University, London.

Parkes, C.M., Benjamin, B. and Fitzgerald, R.G. (1969) Broken heart: a statistical study of increased mortality among widowers. *British Medical Journal*, **1**: 740–743.

Parkin, D.M., Henney, C.R., Quirk, J. and Crooks, J. (1976) Deviations from prescribed treatment after discharge from hospital. *British Medical Journal*, **2**: 686–688.

Parry, O., Platt, S. and Thomson, C. (2000) Out of sight, out of mind: workplace smoking bans and the relocation of smoking at work. *Health Promotion International*, **15**: 125–133.

Pearlin, L.I., Turner, H. and Semple, S. (1989) Coping and the mediation of caregiver stress. In: *Alzheimer's Disease Treatment and Family Stress: Directions for research* (eds E. Light and B.D. Lebowitz). DHSS Publication No. ADM 89–1569. US Government Printing Office, Washington, DC.

Pendleton, D.A. and Bochner, S. (1980) The communication of medical information in general practice consultations as a function of patients' social class. *Social Science and Medicine*, **14A**: 669–673.

Perl, E.R. and Kruger, L. (1996) Nocioception and pain: evolution of concepts and observations. In: *Pain and Touch* (ed. L. Kruger). Academic Press, San Diego, CA.

Perry, A.R. and Baldwin, D.A. (2000) Further evidence of associations of type A personality scores and driving-related attitudes and behaviors. *Perceptual Motor Skills*, **91**: 147–154.

Pert, C.B. and Snyder, S.H. (1973) Opiate receptor: demonstration in nervous tissue. *Science*, **179**: 1011–1014.

Pert, C.B., Dreher, H.E. and Ruff, M.R. (1998) The psychosomatic network: foundations of mind-body medicine. *Alternative Therapies in Health and Medicine*, **4**: 30–41.

Pettingale, K.W., Morris, T., Greer, S. and Haybittle, J.L. (1985) Mental attitudes to cancer: an additional prognostic factor. *Lancet*, **1**: 750.

Petty, R.E. and Cacioppo, J.T. (1981) *Attitudes and Persuasion: Classic and contemporary approaches*. William C. Brown, Dubuque, IO.

Pinfold, J.V. (1999) Analysis of different communication channels for promoting hygiene behaviour. *Health Education Research*, **14**: 629–639.

Pitts, M. and Phillips, K. (1998) *The Psychology of Health: An introduction*. Routledge, London.

Plummer, K. (1988) Organizing AIDS. In: *Social Aspects of AIDS* (eds P. Aggleton and H. Homans). Falmer Press, Lewes, East Sussex: pp. 22–51.

Porter, J. and Jick, H. (1980) Addiction rate in patients treated with narcotics. *New England Journal of Medicine*, **302**: 123.

Povey, R., Conner, M., Sparks, P. *et al.* (2000) Application of the theory of planned behaviour to two dietary behaviours: role of perceived control and efficacy. *British Journal of Health Psychology*, **5**: 121–139.

Quirk, M., Godkin, M. and Schwenzfeier, E. (1993) Evaluation of two AIDS prevention interventions for inner-city adolescents and young adult women. *American Journal of Preventative Medicine*, **9**: 21–26.

Radley, A. (1994) *Making Sense of Illness: The social psychology of health and disease*. Sage, London.

Rahe, R.H. (1968) Life change measurement as a predictor of illness. *Proceedings of the Royal Society of Medicine*, **61**: 124–126.

Rainville, P., Duncan, G.H., Price, D.D. *et al.* (1997) Pain affect encoded in human anterior cingulated but not somatosensory cortex. *Science*, **277**: 968–971.

Ramachandran, V.S. (1993) Behavioral and magnetoencephalic correlates of plasticity in the adult human brain. *Proceedings of the National Academy of Sciences of the USA*, **90**: 20.

Range, L.M. and Calhoun, L.G. (1990) Responses following suicide and other types of death: the perspective of the bereaved. *Omega*, **21**: 311–320.

Reddy, C.V. (1989) Parents' beliefs about vaccination. *British Medical Journal*, **299**: 739.

Redman, S., Webb, G.R., Hennrikus, D.J. *et al.* (1991) The effects of gender on diagnosis of psychological disturbance. *Journal of Behavioral Medicine*, **14**: 527–540.

Reed, G.M., Kemeny, M.E., Taylor, S.E. and Visscher, B.R. (1999) Negative HIV-specific expectancies and AIDS-related bereavement as predictors of symptom onset in asymptomatic HIV-positive gay men. *Health Psychology*, **18**: 354–363.

Reynolds, D.V. (1969) Surgery in the rat during electrical analgesia induced by focal brain stimulation. *Science*, **164**: 444–445.

Rhodewalt, F. and Zone, J.B. (1989) Appraisal of life change, depression and illness in hardy and non-hardy women. *Journal of Personality and Social Psychology*, **56**: 81–88.

Rice, G.E. and Okun, M.A. (1994) Older readers' processing of medical information that contradicts their beliefs. *Journal of Gerontology*, **49**: 119–128.

Richwald, G.A., Wamsley, M.A., Coulson, A.H. and Moriskey, D.E. (1988) Are condom instructions readable? Results of a reliability survey. *Public Health Reports*, **103**: 355–359.

Rimer, B.K., Trock, B., Lermon, C. and King, E. (1991) Why do some women get regular mammograms? *American Journal of Preventative Medicine*, **7**: 69–74.

Roberts, W.C., Wurtele, S.K., Boone, R.R. *et al.* (1981) Reduction of medical fears by use of modelling: a preventative application in a general population of children. *Journal of Pediatric Psychology*, **6**: 203 300.

Rogers, C. (1961) *On Becoming a Person: A therapist's view of psychotherapy.* Houghton-Mifflin, Boston, MA.

Rogers, R.W. (1975) A protection motivation theory of fear appeals and attitude change. *Journal of Psychology*, **91**: 93–114.

Ronis, D.L. (1992) Conditional health threats: Health beliefs, decisions and behaviors among adults. *Health Psychology*, **11**: 127–134.

Rorer, B., Tucker, C.M. and Blake, H. (1988) Long-term nurse-patient interactions: factors in patient compliance or noncompliance to dietary regimen. *Health Psychology*, **7**: 35–46.

Rosenman, R.H., Brand, R.J., Jenkins, C.D. *et al.* (1975) Coronary heart disease in the Western Collaborative Group Study: final follow-up experience of eight and a half years. *Journal of the American Medical Association*, **223**: 872–877.

Rosenstock, I.M. (1966) Why people use health services. *Millbank Memorial Fund Quarterly*, **44**: 94–124.

Ross, C.E. and Mirowsky, J. (1979) A comparison of life-event weighting schemes: change, undesirability, and effect-proportional indices. *Journal of Health and Social Behavior*, **20**: 166–177.

Ross, M. and Olson, J.M. (1981) An expectancy–attribution model of the effects of placebos. *Psychological Review*, **88**: 408–437.

Roter, D.L. and Hall, J.A. (1992) *Doctors Talking with Patients/Patients Talking with Doctors.* Auburn House, Westport, CT.

Roter, D., Lipkin, M. and Korsgaard, A. (1991) Sex differences in patients' and physicians' communication during primary care medical visits. *Medical Care*, **29**: 1083–1093.

Roth, H.P. (1987) Measurement of compliance. *Patient Education and Counselling*, **10**: 107–116.

Rotter, J.B. (1966) Generalised expectancies for internal versus external control of reinforcement. *Psychological Monographs*, **80**(1, no. 609).

Royal College of Surgeons (2003) Communication Skills Initiative. Available on line at: www.rcseng.ac.uk.

Rutter, D.R. (2000) Attendance and reattendance for breast cancer screening: a prospective 3-year test of the theory of planned behaviour. *British Journal of Health Psychology*, **5**: 1–13.

Salmon, P. (2000) *Psychology of Medicine and Surgery.* John Wiley, Chichester.

Sanders, T. and Skevington, S. (2003) Do bowel cancer patients participate in treatment decision-making? Findings from a qualitative study. *European Journal of Cancer Care*, **12**: 166–175.

Sauser, W.L., Arauz, C.G. and Chambers, R.M. (1978) Exploring the relationship between level of office noise and salary recommendations: a preliminary research note. *Journal of Management*, **4**: 57–63.

Savage, R. and Armstrong, D. (1990) Effect of a general practitioner's consulting style on patients' satisfaction: a controlled study, *British Medical Journal*, **301**: 968–970.

Schifter, D.E. and Ajzen, I. (1985) Intention, perceived control, and weight loss: an application of the theory of planned behavior. *Journal of Personality and Social Psychology*, **49**: 843–851.

Schleifer, S.J., Keller, S.E., Camerino, M. *et al.* (1983) Suppression of lymphocyte stimulation following bereavement. *Journal of the American Medical Association*, **250**: 374–377.

Schleifer, S.J., Bhardwaj, S., Lebovits, A., Tanaka, J.S., Messe, M. and Strain, J.J. (1991) Predictors of physician non-adherence to chemotherapy regimens. *Cancer*, **67**: 945–951.

Schwarz, M., Chiang, S., Mueller, N. and Ackenheil, M. (2001) T-helper-1 and T-helper-2 responses in psychiatric disorders. *Brain, Behavior and Immunity*, **15**: 340–370.

Sciacchitano, M., Goldstien, M.B. and DiPlacido, J. (2001) Stress, burnout and hardiness in R.T.s. *Radiology Technology*, **72**: 321–328.

Sclafani, A. and Springer, D. (1976) Dietary obesity in adult rats: similarities to hypothalamic and human obesity. *Physiology and Behavior*, **17**: 461–471.

Scrimshaw, S.M., Engle, P.L. and Zambrana, R.E. (1983) *Prenatal Anxiety and Birth Outcome in US Latinas: Implications for psychosocial interventions.* Paper presented at the annual meeting of the American Psychological Association, Anaheim, CA.

Seidell, J.C. and Rissenen, A.M. (1998) Time trends in world-wide prevalence of obesity. In: *Handbook of Obesity* (eds G.A. Bray, C. Bouchard and W.P.T. James). Marcel Dekker, New York.

Seligman, M.E.P. and Visintainer, M.A. (1985) Turnout rejection and early experience of uncontrollable shock in the rat. In: *Affect Conditioning and Cognition: Essays on the determinants of behavior* (eds F.R. Brush and J.B. Overmier). Lawrence Erlbaum, Hillsdale, NJ.

Sellwood, W. and Tarrier, N. (1994) Demographic factors associated. with extreme non-compliance in schizophrenia. *Social Psychiatry and Psychiatric Epidemiology*, **29**: 172–177.

Selye, H. (1947) *Textbook of Endocrinology.* University of Montreal, Montreal, Quebec.

Serdula, M.K., Collins, M.E., Williamson, D.F. *et al.* (1993) Weight control practices of US adolescents and adults. *Annals of Internal Medicine*, **119**: 667–671.

Shanfield, S.B., Swain, B.J. and Benjamin, G.A.H. (1987) Parents' responses to the death of adult children from accidents and cancer: a comparison. *Omega*, **17**: 289–297.

Shapiro, A.K. (1964) Factors contributing to the placebo effect: their implications for psychotherapy. *American Journal of Psychotherapy*, **18**: 73–88.

Sherbourne, C.D., Hays, R.D., Ordway, L., DiMatteo, M.R. and Kravitz, R.L. (1992) Antecedents of adherence to medical recommendations: results from the Medical Outcomes Study. *Journal of Behavioral Medicine*, **15**: 447–468.

Sherman, J.E. and Liebeskind, J.C. (1980) An endorphinergic centrifugal substrate of pain modulation: recent findings, current concepts, and complexities. In: *Pain* (ed. J.J. Bonica). Raven Press, New York.

Sherman, R.A., Katz, J., Marbach, J.J. and Heermann-Do, K. (1997) Locations, characteristics, and descriptions. In: *Phantom Pain* (ed. R.A. Sherman). Plenum Press, New York.

Sherwood, R.J. (1983) Compliance behavior of hemodialysis patients and the role of the family. *Family Systems Medicine*, **1**: 60–72.

Shillitoe, R.W. (1988) *Psychology and Diabetes: Psychosocial factors in management and control.* Chapman & Hall, London.

Siegel, J.M. and Kuykendall, D.H. (1990) Loss, widowhood, and psychological distress among the elderly. *Journal of Consulting and Clinical Psychology*, **58**: 519–524.

Simkins, L. and Ebenhage, M. (1984) Attitudes towards AIDS, herpes II and toxic shock syndrome, *Psychological Reports*, **55**: 779–786.

Sims, E.A.H. and Horton, E.S. (1968) Endocrine and metabolic adaptation to obesity and starvation. *American Journal of Clinical Nutrition*, **21**: 1455–1470.

Slenker, S.E. and Grant, M.C. (1989) Attitudes, beliefs and knowledge about mammography among women over forty years of age. *Journal of Cancer Education*, **4**: 61–65.

Smetana, J.G. and Alder, N.E. (1980) Fishbein's Value x Expectancy Model: an examination of some assumptions. *Personality and Social Psychology Bulletin*, **6**. 89–96.

Smith, G.B. (1993) Homophobia and attitudes toward gay men and lesbians by psychiatric nurses. *Archives of Psychiatric Nursing*, **7**: 377–384.

Sodroski, J.G., Rosen, C.A. and Haseltine, W.A. (1984) Trans-acting transcription of the long terminal repeat of human T lymphocyte viruses in infected cells. *Science*, **225**: 381–385.

Soendergaard, H.P. and Theorell, T. (2003) A longitudinal study of hormonal reactions accompanying life events in recently resettled refugees. *Psychotherapy and Psychosomatics*, **72**: 49–58.

Soukup, J.E. (1996) *Alzheimer's Disease: A guide to diagnosis, treatment, and management.* Praeger, Westport, CT.

Spanos, N.P., Barber, T.X. and Lang, G. (1974) Effects of hypnotic induction, suggestions of anaesthesia and demands for honesty on subjective reports of pain. In: *Thought and Feeling: Cognitive alternation of feeling states* (eds H. Condon and R.E. Nisbett). Aldine Press, Chicago, IL.

Spinetta, J.J. (1974) The dying child's awareness of death: a review. *Psychological Bulletin*, **81**: 256–260.

Steptoe, A. and Wardle, J. (2001) Locus of control and health behaviour revisited: a multivariate analysis of young adults from 18 countries. *British Journal of Psychology*, **92**: 659–672.

Stewart, M. (1984) Patient characteristics which are related to the doctor–patient interaction. *Family Practice*, **1**: 30–36.

Straneva, P.A., Maxiner, W., Light, K.C. *et al.* (2002) Menstrual cycle, beta-endorphins, and pain sensitivity in premenstrual dysphoric disorder. *Health Psychology*, **21**: 358–367.

Stratton, P. and Hayes, N. (1988) *A Student's Dictionary of Psychology*. Edward Arnold, London.

Strecher, V.J. and Rosenstock, I.M. (1997) The health belief model. In: *Cambridge Handbook of Psychology, Health and Medicine* (eds A. Baum, S. Newman, J. Weinman *et al.*). Cambridge University Press, Cambridge: pp. 113–116.

Strecher, V.J., Champion, V.L. and Rosenstock, I.M. (1997) The health belief model and health behavior. In: *Handbook of Health Behavior Research I: Personal and Social Determinants* (ed. D.S. Gochman). Plenum Press, New York: pp. 71–91.

Streltzer, J. (1997) Pain. In: *Culture and Pathology: A guide to clinical assessment* (eds W.S. Tseng and J. Streltzer). Brunner/Mazel, New York.

Strickland, B.R. (1978) Internal–external expectancies and health-related behaviors. *Journal of Consulting and Clinical Psychology*, **46**: 1192–1211.

Stroebe, W. (2000) *Social Psychology and Health*. Open University Press, Buckingham.

Stroebe, M.S. and Stroebe, W. (1983) Who suffers more? Sex differences in health risks of the widowed. *Psychological Bulletin*, **93**: 279–301.

Stroebe, N. and Stroebe, M. (1987) *Bereavement and Health*. Cambridge University Press, New York.

Stunkard A.J. (1988) Some perspectives on human obesity: Its causes. *Bulletin of the New York Academy of Medicine*, **64**: 902–923.

Stunkard, A.J., Sørensen, T.I.A., Hanis, C. *et al.* (1986) An adoption study of human obesity. *New England Journal of Medicine*, **314**: 193–198.

Swerdlow, N.R., Geyer, M.A., Vale, W.W. and Koob, G.F. (1986) Corticotropin releasing factor potentiates acoustic startle in rats: blockade by chlordiazepoxide. *Psychopharmacology*, **88**: 147–152.

Taffinder, N.J., McManus, I.C., Gul, Y. *et al.* (1998) Effect of sleep deprivation on surgeons' dexterity on laparoscopy simulator. *Lancet*, **352**: 1191.

Talbott, E.O., Findlay, R.C., Kuller, L.H. *et al.* (1990) Noise-induced hearing loss and blood pressure. *Journal of Occupational Medicine*, **32**: 690–697.

Tanner, E.K.W. and Feldman, R.H.L. (1997) Strategies for enhancing appointment keeping in low-income chronically ill clients. *Nursing Research*, **46**: 342–344.

Taylor, S.E. (1983) Adjusting to threatening events: a theory of cognitive adaptation. *American Psychologist*, **38**: 1161–1173.

Taylor, S.E. (1995) *Health Psychology*. McGraw-Hill, New York.

Tedesco, L.A., Keffer, M.A. and Fleck-Kandath, C. (1991) Self-efficacy, reasoned action, and oral health behavior reports: a social cognitive approach to compliance. *Journal of Behavioural Medicine*, **14**: 341–355.

Temoshok, L., Sweet, D.M. and Zich, J.A. (1987) A three city comparison of the public's knowledge and attitudes about AIDS. *Psychology and Health*, **1**: 43–60.

Theorell, T., Lind, E. and Floderus, B. (1975) The relationship of disturbing life changes and emotion to the early development of myocardial infarction and other serious illnesses. *International Journal of Epidemiology*, **4**: 281–293.

Thomas, V.J., Dixon, A.L. and Milligan, P. (1999) Cognitive-behaviour therapy for the management of sickle cell disease pain: an evaluation of a community-based intervention. *British journal of Health Psychology*, **4**: 209–229.

Totman, R.G. (1976) Cognitive dissonance and the placebo response. *European Journal of Social Psychology*, **5**: 119–125.

Totman, R. G. (1987) *The Social Causes of Illness*. Souvenir Press, London.

Treisman, A.M. (1964) Verbal cues, language and meaning in selective attention. *American Journal of Psychology*, **77**: 206–219.

Tulving, E. (1974) Cue-dependent forgetting. *American Scientist*, **62**: 74–82.

Turk, D.C., Meichenbaum, D.H. and Berman, W. (1979) Application of biofeedback for the regulation of pain: a critical review. *Psychological Bulletin*, **86**: 1322–1338.

Turk, D.C., Meichenbaum, D. and Genest, M. (1983) *Pain and Behavioral Medicine: A cognitive–behavioral perspective*. Guilford Press, New York.

Turner, J. and Wheaton, B. (1995) Checklist measurement of stressful life events. In: *Measuring Stress* (eds S. Cohen, R.C. Kessler and L. Underwood Gordon). Oxford University Press, New York: pp. 29–58.

Tyler, P.A., Carroll, D. and Cunningham, S.E. (1991) Stress and well-being in nurses: a comparison of the public and private sectors. *International Journal of Nursing Studies*, **28**: 125–130.

Valente, S.M. (2003) Aftermath of a patient's suicide: a case study. *Perspectives in Psychiatric Care*, **39**: 17–22.

Varni, J.W., Thompson, K.L. and Hanson, V. (1987) The Varni–Thompson Paediatric Pain Questionnaire: I. Chronic musculo-skeletal pain in juvenile rheumatoid arthritis. *Pain*, **28**: 27–38.

Vertefeuille, J., Marx, M.A., Tun, W. *et al.* (2000) Decline in self-reported high-risk injection-related behaviors among HIV-seropositive participants in the Baltimore needle exchange program. *AIDS and Behavior*, **4**: 381–388.

Vinar, O. (1969) Dependence on a placebo: a case report. *British Journal of Psychiatry*, **115**: 1189–1190.

Vincent, P. (1971) Factors influencing patient noncompliance: a theoretical approach. *Nursing Resesarch*, **20**: 509–516.

Vincent, C.A. (1989) A controlled study of the treatment of migraine by acupuncture. *Clinical Journal of Pain*, **5**: 305–312.

Von Frey, M. (1895) *Untersuchungen über der menschlichen Haut. Erste Abhandlung: Druckempfindung und Schmerz.* Hirzel, Leipzig.

Wadden, T.A. and Anderton, C.H. (1982) The clinical use of hypnosis. *Psychological Bulletin*, **91**: 215–243.

Wadden, T.A. and Brownwell, K.D. (1984) The development and modification of dietary practices in individuals. In: *Behavioral Health: A handbook of health enhancement and disease prevention* (eds J.D. Matarazzo, S.M. Weiss, J.A. Herd *et al.*). John Wiley, New York.

Waitzkin, H. (1985) Information giving in medical care. *Journal of Health and Social Behavior*, **26**: 81–101.

Walker, J. (2001) *Control and the Psychology of Health*. Open University Press, Buckingham.

Wall, P.D. and Jones, M. (1991) *Defeating Pain: The war against a silent epidemic.* Plenum Press, New York.

Wallston, K.A., Walston, B.S. and DeVellis, R. (1978) Development of the Multidimensional Health Locus of Control (MHLC) scale. *Health Education Monographs*, **6**: 5–25.

Walter, T., Littlewood, J. and Pickering, M. (2000) Death in the news: the public investigation of private emotion. In: *Death, Dying and Bereavement* (eds D. Dickenson, M. Johnson and J.S. Katz). Sage/Open University, London.

Warner, K.E. (1977) The effects of the anti-smoking campaign on cigarette smoking. *American Journal of Public Health*, **67**: 645–650.

Warner, K.E. and Murt, H.A. (1982) Impact of the anti-smoking campaign on smoking prevalence: A cohort analysis. *Journal of Public Health Policy*, **3**: 374–390.

Weisman, C.S. and Teitelbaum, M.A. (1989) Women and health care communication. *Patient Education and Counselling*, **13**: 183–199.

West, C. (1984) When the doctor is a 'lady': Power, status, and gender in physician-patient encounters. *Symbolic Interaction*, **7**: 87–106.

Wing, R.R., Epstein, L.H., Nowalk, M.P. and Lamparski, D.M. (1986) Behavioral self-regulation in the treatment of patients with diabetes mellitus. *Psychological Bulletin*, **99**: 78–89.

Winzelberg, A.J., Eppstein, D., Eldredge, K.L. *et al.* (2000) Effectiveness of an internet-based program for reducing risk factors for eating disorders. *Journal of Consulting and Clinical Psychology*, **68**: 346–350.

Wiseman, C.V., Gray, J.J., Moismann, J.E. and Ahrens, A.H. (1992) Cultural expectations of thinness in women: An update. *International Journal of Eating Disorders*, **11**: 85–89.

Wolf, S.L., Nacht, M. and Kelly, J.L. (1982) EMG feedback training during dynamic movement for low back pain patients. *Behavior Therapy*, **13**: 395–406.

Wolpe, J. (1958) *Psychotherapy by Reciprocal Inhibition*. Stanford University Press, Stanford, CA.

Woodcock, A., Stenner, K. and Ingram, R. (1992) Young people talking about HIV and AIDS: Interpretations of personal risk of infection. *Health Education Research: Theory and Practice*, **7**: 229–247.

Worden, J.W. (1991) *Grief Counseling and Grief Therapy: A handbook for the mental health practitioner*. Springer, New York.

World Health Organization (1993) *Doctor–Patient Interaction and Communication*. WHO, Geneva.

Wortman, C.B. and Silver, R.L. (1987) Coping with irrevocable loss. In: *Cataclysms, Crises and Catastrophes: Psychology in action* (eds G. Vandenbos and B. Bryant). American Psychological Association, Washington, DC.

Wysocki, T., Green, L. and Huxtable, K.(1989) Blood glucose monitoring by diabetic adolescents: compliance and metabolic control. *Health Psychology*, **8**: 267–284.

Yapko, M.D. (1995) *Essential Hypnosis*. Brunner/Mazel, New York.

Yinon, Y. and Bizman, A. (1980) Noise, success and failure as determinants of helping behaviour. *Personality and Social Psychology Bulletin*, **6**: 125–130.

Yoast, R., Williams, M.A., Deitchman, S.D. and Champion, H.C. (2001) Report of the Council on Scientific Affairs: Methadone maintenance and needle-exchange programs to reduce the medical and public health consequences of drug abuse. *Journal of Addictive Diseases*, **20**: 15–40.

Yoong, A.F.E., Lim, J., Hudson, C.N. and Chard, T. (1992) Audit of compliance with antenatal protocols. *British Medical Journal*, **305**: 1184–1186.

Zautra, A.J. (1998) Arthritis: behavioral and psychosocial aspects. In: *Behavioral Medicine and Women: A comprehensive handbook* (eds E.A. Blechman and K.D. Brownell). Guilford Press, New York: pp. 554–558.

Zborowski, M. (1952) Cultural components in response to pain. *Journal of Social Issues*, **8**: 16–30.

Zisook, S., Peterkin, J.J., Schuchter, S.R. and Bardone, A. (1995) Death, dying and bereavement. In: *Managing Chronic Illness: A biological perspective* (eds P.M. Nicassio and T.W. Smith). American Psychological Association, Washington, DC.

Zola, I.K. (1966) Culture and symptoms – an analysis of patients' presenting complaints. *American Sociological Review*, **31**: 615–630.

Appendix

Answers to rapid recap questions

Chapter 1

1. What is the communication cycle?

1. The process by which we communicate. A message is transmitted from one person (the sender) to another (the recipient) and the cycle is completed by feedback from the recipient back to the sender.

2. What is meant by 'patient-centred' and 'doctor-centred' approaches to interaction?

2. Patient-centred means treating the patient as an individual, rather than a commodity. The patient is an active participant in the interaction and can influence the outcome. Doctor-centred means the practitioner asking the patient questions about their condition, which allows the provision of a diagnosis and appropriate treatment. Communication is two-way but is directed by one of the participants.

3. What does the acronym SOLER stand for?

3. Face one another **S**quarely
   Have an **O**pen posture
   Lean slightly towards the other person
   Maintain good **E**ye contact
   Try to **R**elax but pay attention

Chapter 2

1. Identify the key elements in the theory of planned behaviour.

1. The theory of planned behaviour proposes that actions, such as health behaviours, are determined by a combination of behavioural intention (deciding to achieve a goal) and perceived behavioural control (believing that you can or cannot perform a behaviour).

2. The following factors could affect an individual who is thinking about giving up smoking: the existence of many non-smoking restaurants; the belief that smoky clothes are unpleasant; a desire to combat the effects of smoking on their asthma; the knowledge that they can stop themselves from starting again once they have said they've given up. Explain which of these factors would relate to each aspect of the theory of planned behaviour.

2. Behavioural intention – the existence of many non-smoking restaurants; the belief that smoky clothes are unpleasant; desire to combat the effects of smoking on their asthma.

   Perceived behavioural control – the knowledge that they can stop themselves from starting again once they have said they've given up.

Chapter 3

1. What are the three factors that affect compliance to medical advice according to Ley's model?

1. a. Understanding
   b. Memory
   c. Satisfaction.

2. Identify four factors that could affect a patient's ability to recall information they have been given.

2. a. Four from:
   Anxiety – more anxious patients seem to have better recall
   Medical knowledge – patients with greater knowledge have better recall
   Primacy effect – patients have better recall for the first information presented to them
   Importance – statements perceived by the patient to be important are recalled better

Volume of information – when more information is presented, more is recalled but the percentage remembered is lower.

3. Describe three ways that a health professional could improve adherence by changing the way spoken information is presented to patients.

3. a. Understanding – e.g. by avoiding jargon or using shorter sentences
    b. Satisfaction – e.g. by using a more patient-centred communication style
    c. Memory – e.g. by summarising/repeating key information, saying the most important things first and presenting small amounts of information or presenting information slowly.

Chapter 4

1. Describe the three stages of the general adaptation syndrome.

1. a. Alarm reaction – the body's mechanisms for dealing with danger are activated
    b. Resistance stage – the person struggles to cope with the stress, and the body attempts to return to its previous physiological state
    c. Exhaustion stage – if the stressor persists and the body cannot return to its previous state, physical resources become depleted, eventually leading to collapse.

2. Why might people with type A personalities be at greater risk from stress?

2. People with type A personalities tend to be highly competitive, aggressive, impatient and hostile, with a strong urge for success. Their behaviour tends to be goal-directed and performed at speed. With these types of personality factor, such people are more likely to suffer from stress as they tend to put themselves in more stressful situations. Alternatively, another biological factor may be responsible for both type A personalities and increased susceptibility to the effects of stress.

3. a. What is meant by emotion-focused and problem-focused coping strategies?

3. a. Emotion-focused coping strategies aim to manage the negative effects on the individual, for example by keeping busy to take one's mind off the problem, preparing oneself for the worst, praying for strength and guidance, ignoring the situation in the belief that the problem will go away, or bottling feelings up. Problem-focused

coping strategies aim to reduce the causes of stress, for example by discussing the situation with a professional, relying on one's own past experiences to tackle the issue or dealing with the situation one step at time.

b. Which coping strategies, emotion-focused or problem-focused, are more effective in general?

b. Problem-focused strategies are more effective because they deal with the cause of the stress.

c. In what situations would emotion-focused strategies be more beneficial than problem-focused ones?

c. When it is beyond the scope of the individual to effect change.

Chapter 5

1. Describe one way in which pain is measured in a clinical setting and one way in which it can be measured for the purposes of research.

1. Clinical setting: Self-reporting, where the patient records their pain in words as a description or on a diagram, indicating the location and intensity

    Research: Cold-pressor test, where the participant has to keep their hand submerged in ice cold water for as long as they can, the time elapsed before the hand is removed indicating their pain tolerance.

2. Too much work on a computer or reading a book can lead to an eye-strain headache. How would the gate control theory of pain account for the effectiveness of rubbing one's eyes to relieve the pain?

2. The physical effect of rubbing the eyes stimulates the large (A-beta) nerve fibres that send signals up to the gate in the spinal cord and close it. This prevents perception of the pain of the headache.

3. Vinar (1969) reported a case study of an individual who had become dependent upon a placebo. Use the idea of expectation to explain how this situation might have arisen.

3. The belief that a treatment will relieve pain results in pain reduction. If the patient had been taking the placebo for a long time and had not experienced pain (because it was no longer necessary) they could have built up an expectation that they would

suffer if they stopped taking it. The patient's absence of pain while taking the placebo would have confirmed their belief that they needed it to be pain-free.

Chapter 6

1. **How does the idea proposed by Worden (1991) differ from the stage processes described by Kübler-Ross and Parkes and why might Worden's approach be more useful?**

1. By stating that it is more useful to identify the tasks to be achieved through mourning:
   - Accepting the reality of the loss
   - Working through the pain
   - Adjusting to the absence of the deceased from the environment
   - Moving forward in life.

   Worden's approach might be more useful because it allows for individual differences that will arise in the exact stages or feelings that each person experiences and the order in which they happen.

2. **a. Identify four differences between the grieving of men and women.**

2. a. Four from:
   Women tend to display more overt grief than men
   Women are more likely to suffer obsessional grief
   Women are more likely to benefit from attending a funeral
   Women are less likely to turn to alcohol than men
   Women describe feelings of abandonment whereas men describe feeling dismembered
   Women tend to feel angry and cry whereas men feel 'choked up' and guilty

Men make a faster social recovery than women but take longer to overcome the emotional consequences.

b. **Will all men and women differ in these ways?**

b. No, there will be individual, cultural and societal differences as well as gender-related ones.

c. **In what ways is the experience of bereaved children similar to and different from that of adults?**

c. Bereaved children suffer many of the same emotions, of guilt, anger, numbness and depression as adults. However they differ from adults in their less predictable response and their differing understanding of the concept of death, depending on their age.

3. **The problem pages of magazines often describe the misery of people who care for a relative with a progressive disease, such as multiple sclerosis, who feel as though they are grieving before their relative has even died. How would you explain what they were experiencing if you were asked to do so by a hospital visitor expressing similar concerns?**

3. I would explain that they are experiencing anticipatory grieving. They identify feelings of loss that resemble bereavement while the individual is still alive because the person they once knew no longer exists. They may experience anger, fear of abandonment as the relationship deteriorates, depression and sleeplessness. Anticipatory grief can also lead to an increased risk of catching infections but if carers themselves have good social support, they tend to cope better. In addition, emotions including sadness, feeling overwhelmed or trapped, frustration and guilt may be felt. These will be distressing but are common in this situation.

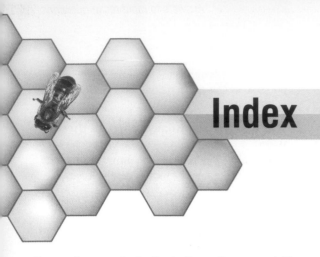

Index

Page references in *italics* indicate figures and illustrations and those in **bold** indicate tables